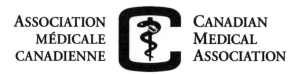

ASSOCIATION
MÉDICALE
CANADIENNE

CANADIAN
MEDICAL
ASSOCIATION

The Pain Relief Handbook

Dr. Chris Wells and Graham Nown

KEY PORTER BOOKS

Copyright © 1998 by Chris Wells and Graham Nown
First published in the United Kingdom by Ebury Press

All rights reserved. No part of this work covered by the copyrights
hereon may be reproduced or used in any form or by any means –
graphic, electronic or mechanical, including photocopying, recording,
taping or information storage and retrieval systems – without the prior
written permission of the publisher, or in the case of photocopying or
other reprographic copying, a licence from the Canadian Copyright
Licensing Agency.

Canadian Cataloguing in Publication Data

Wells, Chris
    The pain relief handbook

(Your personal health series)
Canadian ed.
Includes index.
ISBN 1-55013-945-2

1. Chronic pain – Treatment.   2. Chronic pain – Popular works.
I. Nown, Graham.   II. Title. III. Series

RB127.W44   1998   616'.0472   C97-932694-X

THE CANADA COUNCIL | LE CONSEIL DES ARTS
    FOR THE ARTS | DU CANADA
    SINCE 1957 | DEPUIS 1957

The publisher gratefully acknowledges the support of the Canada Council
for the Arts and the Ontario Arts Council for its publishing program.

The statements and opinions expressed herein are those of the authors,
and are not intended to be used as a substitute for consultation with your
physician. All matters pertaining to your health should be directed to a
healthcare professional.

Key Porter Books Limited
70 The Esplanade
Toronto, Ontario
Canada M5E 1R2

Diagrams: Lianne Friesen
Electronic formatting: Heidy Lawrance Associates

Printed and bound in Canada

98 99 00 01 6 5 4 3 2 1

Contents

Foreword

The link between pain and injury seems so obvious that it is widely believed that pain is always the result of physical damage and that the amount of pain we feel is proportional to the severity of the injury. In general, this relationship between pain and injury holds true: a small cut on a finger hurts a little, while a laceration of the skin can be agonizing. However, the relationship is not always so simple. Many forms of chronic pain, such as back aches and muscle pains, show that there is often little or no relationship between pain and injury. The absence of a fixed relationship between pain and injury is also frequently evident in day-to-day events. Research has shown that the amount and quality of pain we feel are also influenced by our previous experiences and how well we remember them, by our ability to understand the cause of the pain and to grasp its consequences. Even the culture in which we have been brought up plays an essential role in how we feel and respond to pain.

Remarkable advances in our understanding of pain and our ability to treat it have occurred in recent years. Yet the layman who wishes to learn about these advances by reading medical journals and books is often deterred by specialized jargon or complicated terminology. On the other hand, facile explanations in the popular media are often suspect because they tend to emphasize the spectacular aspects of research or therapy and ignore the caution that should accompany a newly growing field of research. They thereby mislead or misinform the reader, and frequently hold out promise of panaceas that fail to materialize.

Dr. Wells has written an excellent book that can be recommended to the layman. He presents complex information about pain in a readable, intelligent format, and evaluates the clinical and laboratory research in a fair, balanced manner that evokes the excitement of new discoveries without offering total cures for every kind of pain for everyone. Furthermore, he converses with the reader as a fellow human being concerned about pain and suffering.

Dr. Wells is an internationally known specialist in the field of pain treatment. His considerable experience and knowledge allow him to deal with a wide range of pain problems. However, he has focused on those aspects of pain that are likely to be of most interest to the general reader – the major clinical problems such as back pain, myofascial pain, and headache.

The field of pain is growing rapidly. Dr. Wells has captured the excitement of a growing field in medicine, psychology, nursing and many other health sciences. Anyone who suffers pain, knows other who do, or is simply curious about an important problem in human life will benefit from reading this book.

Ronald Melzack, *Research Director*
McGill – Montreal General Hospital Pain Center
Professor of Pain Studies, McGill University
Montreal, Canada

Publisher's Note

Dr. Chris Wells is the director of the Centre for Pain Relief at Walton Hospital, in Liverpool, England. When he and Dr. Eric Ghadiali established the center's pain management program in 1982, it was the first of its kind in the United Kingdom. The center is internationally famous for its wide range of treatments, and for pioneering many new forms of therapy.

This edition has been comprehensively updated and adapted for North American readers.

Acknowledgments

The authors gratefully acknowledge assistance given by the Pain Relief Research Foundation, Walton Hospital, Liverpool, England; the patients mentioned in this book, some of whose names have been changed; Dr. Eric Ghadiali; Dr. Bill Wiles; dietitian Pat Crooks; all the therapists on the Pain Management Programme; members of Self-Help in Pain; the Arthritis and Rheumatism Council; the Association to Aid the Sexual and Personal Relationships of People with a Disability; Relaxation for Living; Professor Ronald Melzack, for permission to reproduce part of the McGill–Melzack Pain Questionnaire; Dr. John Watson; Sue Corness, for secretarial support.

Medical advisors to the CMA for *The Pain Relief Handbook:*

A.J.M. Clark MD FRCPC
Director, Pain Management Unit
Queen Elizabeth II Health Sciences Centre
Halifax NS

Linda Robinson MD FRCPC
Director, Pain Clinic
Ottawa Civic Hospital, Ottawa ON

Linda Wynne MBBS FRCPC, Ottawa ON

Introduction

It became more than something physical. Rather than taking up the space somewhere between my foot and lower back, the pain took up my whole life. I didn't meet people. I spent a lot of time in bed. It not only took me over, it affected all the people around me...

At some time in our lives we all endure the agony of pain. If we are lucky, it may only be passing. When it persists, it can turn into a primeval monster in our midst, breaking up families, causing depression, financial hardship or divorce.

Prolonged pain has the power to crush our self-confidence and lead us to lose a sense of who we are. It is like being trapped in an endlessly revolving door. At its extreme, sufferers may even be driven to attempt suicide.

As one medical study put it, "Pain is not just an epidemic, but a major social problem." It inflicts terrible damage at a cost that cannot be counted in dollars – disrupting life, destroying relationships, cutting us off from family and friends.

Anyone with a blinding migraine attack or nagging back pain will know that it is impossible to function normally – to concentrate at work, take the kids to the park, watch a movie or enjoy dinner in a restaurant. Pain becomes the center of every working day, shouldering aside everything of value and importance. One patient, John, explained: "I didn't want to do anything. My family life went out of the window. I just sat in a chair like an old zombie. If my grandchildren came to the house, I would vanish upstairs and lie on the bed to get out of the way."

Pain makes demands of us and puts us under pressure. As it progresses, our lives have to be organized around it. Even reality becomes distorted. Here's how it affected Philippa, a photographer suffering from sciatica caused by a slipped disk: "The biggest effect is social isolation. You don't believe you can go out and meet people anymore. You don't believe you have anything to offer them. In a sense, your pain becomes your identity. There is nothing else to speak about. All your experience is about pain and being in bed surrounded by four walls. It becomes a self-perpetuating cycle."

Allowing pain to take us over totally is not unusual. John, who suffers from osteoarthritis, describes how pain changed his outlook: "I didn't want to socialize with people at all. Before my illness I was a friendly, hail-fellow-well-met sort of guy. Then I just withdrew into my shell. The pain was really severe. Because of it, I slowly began to lose the use of the rest of my body."

If any of those symptoms sound familiar, then the chances are that you are suffering from prolonged, or chronic, pain. Eventually, whatever illness you have becomes secondary to the pain itself. In addition you may suffer from loss of sleep, constant tiredness, digestive disorders and drug dependency. As every sufferer knows, the agony of pain is like being on a treadmill. The longer it persists, the more the edges of life become blurred, leaving little hope to cling to.

No Magic Wands, No Magic Pills

Traditional methods of treating chronic or recurrent pain are often ineffectual. It is perhaps not surprising that a 1978 survey of family physicians in the United States revealed that many of them lose interest in those long-term disorders for which pills offer little relief and the chances of successful treatment are slight.

The problem also lies within ourselves. We have been conditioned through advertising, television and magazines to expect a pill for every symptom we suffer. It is not a healthy outlook to have – for us or our society. Medicine may have made great strides, but miracles are not yet in sight.

One of the problems of pain is that it produces a dependence on doctors and drugs. When we sit down in a doctor's office and complain of a headache or backache, what we are really doing is trying to hand over our pain to the doctor and ask him or her to take it away. This brings us to the first rule of pain relief, and it may come as a surprise: *the only effective way to overcome pain is to do something about it ourselves.* Hoping for a medical magic wand to wave it away is not the solution.

Pain researchers find that people who suffer most from chronic pain are those who hand the problem to their doctor and settle for the painkiller-and-rest approach. Those who suffer least are those who exercise regularly, make an effort to change their outlook and place pain low on their scale of importance.

Accepting the burden of your own pain and resolving to do something about it is a big step to take. Some sufferers trail their pain from doctor to doctor and try countless prescriptions in the hope that someone else will take the agony away from them. Others, after years of discomfort, are even reluctant to give up their pain. They can no longer visualize life without it.

Of course it is wonderful news if you can find a painkiller that completely removes the pain and allows you to resume normal living. The sad truth is, however, that life rarely runs so smoothly. It is probably safe to say that most people taking drugs for chronic pain find that the effects of them eventually wear off. It is quite common for pain sufferers to take a dozen or more painkillers a day and still have pain and limited activity. To add to their problems, they will likely have to cope with the unpleasant side effects of withdrawal if they try to discontinue the drugs. Thousands of people find themselves caught in this cruel trap and turn in desperation to different doctors, who in turn offer different drugs.

This lesson underlines that first rule of pain relief: try to do something about it yourself, rather than leave it to others. In the long march of medicine, this is a new concept, but results encourage the view that self-help may be the most hopeful pain treatment of the future.

While it is not advisable to stop any kind of treatment without medical advice, recent pain research has shown that drugs may actually inhibit the body's own ability to get better. Total reliance on drugs is unwise when we have resources within our bodies that may fight pain more effectively, with no unpleasant effects.

One patient, James, described the drawback of drugs: "I have had headaches all my life, but for the past 10 or 11 years they have been almost constant. A pressure pain is with me when I go to bed and it is still there when I wake up in the morning. It is so long since I have been free from pain that I no longer know what it is like to be different. My doctor prescribed tranquilizers, but they just made me very tired. The problem became worse. I was unable to do the things I wanted to do. As a result, my anxiety increased. When I mentioned this to my doctor, he told me to keep taking the tablets. Eventually, I decided to stop. The pain is still there, but I feel more alive as a person. More ready to do something to help myself."

The Scope of the Pain Problem – Some Shocking Statistics

Most people take painkillers when they feel pain. It has been estimated that 70 percent of patients who turn to painkillers still suffer terrible pain. The scope of the problem, and the misery it causes, is now so vast and commonplace that it becomes almost difficult to comprehend.

A health study in Britain revealed that 11.5 percent of the population suffer chronic pain: that is, pain that occurs at some occasion on every day for more than three months. When the survey was carried out among members of the public visiting patients in hospital, 15 percent of the visitors admitted having chronic pain themselves.

Wherever we live and however we live, pain has become a disabling scourge on society. It makes no distinction between white and black, poor and rich. Millions of ordinary people throughout the world suffer silently because they believe nothing can be done to help them. The desperation of one patient, Alan, sums up their feelings: "I was on twenty pills a day," he said, "but nothing was working. I would have tried anything to get rid of the pain. Anything at all."

As many as 30 percent of people in the United States are thought to suffer chronic pain. In fact, more than 50 million Americans are partly or completely disabled by pain for a few days each month – a loss of 700 million working days a year. And some of these people may never recover from it. Add to this the cost of health care bills, compensation payments and, in many cases, attorneys' fees, and the price of pain soars to almost $100 billion a year.

In Britain, the most common symptom doctors have to deal with is headache. About 30 percent of the population suffers from headache at some time during any one year. In North America over 26 million people suffer from migraine headaches, and many have given up seeking help from their doctors.

Twenty-one percent of otherwise healthy people in Britain are said to complain of back pain in any one-month period. According to Britain's Arthritis and Rheumatism Council, back pain accounts for around 20 million lost working days each year. Statistics like these are plentiful: in the U.S. it has been calculated that 5 percent of the cost of a first-class letter goes toward covering the wages of U.S. Postal Service mail carriers off work with back pain.

Pain is the biggest drain on a nation's resources. In the state of Washington, for example, 36 percent of the state's compensation payments go to patients suffering from lower-back pain. In California, hospital treatment for back ailments alone costs around $80 million a year. Figures such as these tell merely a tiny part of the story. Only those who suffer pain – from migraine to backache, from diabetes to dreaded forms of cancer – can truly understand its demoralizing effects.

In Europe and the United States more than 200 times the amount allocated to pain research is spent on painkillers, an annual drug bill of $2 billion in the U.S. alone. However, advances in pain management and research in the past 20 years have proved that relief can be achieved that does not necessarily involve increasing drug dosages or other medical treatments. Learning to cope with pain and increasing our activities, with less reliance on medicine and doctors, are sometimes the best ways forward.

Know about Pain to Conquer It

The first practical step on the road to conquering pain is to understand its nature and the mechanics of how it works.

There are essentially two types of pain. *Acute pain* is the kind of reaction we feel when we burn a finger or drop something heavy on a foot. It is the sensation that makes us jerk our finger from the flame or move away from danger rapidly. Its purpose is to give us useful warning that we have hurt ourselves or suffered tissue damage. We all need acute pain at some time in our lives. It is positive, practical and protective – so much so that it is actually extremely harmful if we are unable to feel it. There are unusual cases of people who do not feel acute pain at all, and someone who has been in severe pain for 20 years might envy them, but they are unfortunate. Without the sensation of acute pain they might be unaware they have a broken limb, or a serious burn that could otherwise have been avoided.

Chronic pain – pain that simply doesn't go away – can have many causes. Often, an accident, injury or some physical reason triggers the pain; this may be untreatable, or treatment may fail. Frequently in chronic pain the amount of discomfort seems to far exceed the physical cause. It is well accepted that chronic pain is an emotional experience, and that psychological factors play a large part in maintaining the discomfort felt.

The chronic-pain sufferer, however, is left with a pain that is both long-term and debilitating. The pain is not useful because it is not an indication of minute-by-minute tissue damage. There is no advantage in sufferers seeking instant medical advice because treatment is not going to cure them. More important, rest and prolonged medication are not going to be helpful either; they are only liable to lead to further problems, rather than resolve the symptoms.

Chronic-pain sufferers may have any one of a dozen or so conditions or diseases. These can range from arthritis and back problems to diabetes, and include a host of other diseases, such as multiple sclerosis or shingles. What they all have in common is that the pain is both long-term and disabling. The most important point to remember about chronic pain is that it serves no useful purpose at all.

The Pain Management Self-Help Program

The self-help pain relief program in this book is based on methods used by the pain relief clinic at Walton Hospital, Liverpool – one of the biggest in the world – and research carried out at the Pain Relief Research Institute adjoining the hospital. The institute is the first of its kind in the world devoted entirely to research into chronic pain in people. It has become

---

Chronic pain and acute pain are different

Dr. Richard Chapman and Dr. John Bonica of the University of Washington School of Medicine did a study on pain and found three important differences between acute and chronic pain:

- mental attitudes play a great part in someone suffering long-term pain;
- surroundings and social relationships affect chronic-pain sufferers more than acute-pain sufferers;
- the link between the source of the pain and the pain itself actually becomes weaker as chronic pain progresses. In other words, the body almost forgets the original illness or injury but continues to generate pain messages. The pain begins almost to acquire a life of its own.

By bearing these points in mind and resolving to work on them by following a pain relief program, you can make great strides toward mastering the pain in your body.

an international focus of pain research, sharing discoveries and passing on training in pain relief techniques.

Twenty-nine percent of people on the pain management self-help program are able to go back to work after previously being unable to work at all. Many more resume an active social life and enjoy the company of family and friends without the demands that pain once placed upon them.

The outpatient program at Walton runs for four weeks and consists of activities and therapies specifically designed to help patients cope better with their pain. It is not a miracle cure and patients are told that it is unlikely their pain will have disappeared by the end of the program. What they may hope to achieve are reduced pain levels and a feeling of being less distressed and restricted by their pain. There is also every hope that they will become more active and confident, less reliant on pills and other physical methods of pain relief, and that they will feel generally better and more in control.

Most people who come to the pain relief clinic view it as a last resort. Often, they have seen several doctors and received a variety of drugs, with little success. If their pain had had one simple cause, it would have been treated and cured long ago. As for many chronic-pain sufferers who have found no relief, pain for these people has become a complex process that responds more readily to the range of therapies offered in the program. For them, there is no other treatment, long-term, that is likely to work. It is a last opportunity to gain control over their pain and improve the quality of their lives.

The steps outlined in the following chapters can help you develop the same ability to cope with long-term pain through physical and mental exercise.

Chronic pain has very important psychological as well as physical aspects. What you think about, how you behave, how other people treat you, your attitudes and feelings can *all* exert very strong influences on your perception of pain. These psychological aspects can act almost like a volume control, turning the volume up or down on the pain, depending on what you are thinking about or doing.

This "behavioral" approach to pain management concentrates on the psychological rather than the physical aspects of pain, and provides an effective way of helping many people who suffer with chronic pain.

Treatment is provided by a multidisciplinary team of professionals, including medical staff, a clinical psychologist, occupational therapists, physiotherapists, a dance instructor, a dietician, a tai chi instructor, a healer, voluntary workers and "pain graduates" – people who have successfully completed the program and return to provide extra assistance. All members of the team have extensive experience in the management and treatment of chronic pain. (Pain relief clinics like this one, which provide a multidisciplinary approach to the treatment of pain, are available in Canada, and the United States has many such facilities. Physicians outside such clinics may still draw upon other disciplines in the long-term management of chronic-pain patients.)

Self-Help Pain Management Aims
The aims of the program, reflected in this book, are to
  1. increase the daily activities of chronic-pain sufferers;
  2. increase physical fitness: power, endurance and flexibility;
  3. teach relaxation skills;
  4. reduce distress and disability;
  5. increase self-confidence and the ability to function, and improve coping skills;
  6. eliminate unhelpful beliefs about pain;

7. reduce addictive or unnecessary drugs;
8. improve understanding of pain;
9. improve sleep and reduce the use of sedatives;
10. eliminate aids, such as braces, canes, collars and wheel-chairs;
11. allow a return to work where appropriate;
12. reduce dependence on doctors and the health care system.

Pain is expensive, in both personal terms and the welfare of society. But the price is high only until you do something about it yourself. Once that decision is made, work, family and personal relationships become a possibility again. In the words of Margaret, a car crash victim: "I have realized that my life has not come to an end. There are all kinds of things I can do and goals I can achieve. I can cope with the pain by removing myself from it. I am no longer a prisoner. For the first time, I have a sense of freedom."

Breaking the chains of pain is not easy. It requires patience, perseverance and a regular program. But improving the quality of life and picking up again at the point where pain took over are not impossible. The voice of another patient sums it up: "I used to creak around a whole lot. Now I've got muscles that are working again. The pain is still there, but I can ignore it. I'm not aware of it and I think it's getting less. My life goes on as normal."

By understanding more about your own pain and the potential within you to conquer it, you may be able to share this confidence.

How to Use This Book
Many people with chronic pain feel jaded, and may want to get straight to the exercises, relaxation training and ways of

coping that we outline. In that case, read chapters 4, 5 and 6, and get started. Read chapters 3, 7 and 10 to keep the routine going, and build up your knowledge about pain with the remaining chapters.

ONE

How Pain Works

There was a time when bearing pain was thought of as something noble or character building. From biblical days through to the Victorian era, withstanding pain was seen to be somehow admirable or meritorious. Happily, it was one Victorian attitude Queen Victoria herself did not share. Her subjects may have felt that there should be no relief of labor pain, but when Victoria found herself pregnant, the adage "In sorrow shalt thou bring forth children" went out of the window. The queen pioneered anesthesia *à la reine* when she had pain relief during childbirth.

Her decision helped to outmode the idea that bearing pain is somehow heroic or necessary. We now know that long-term pain is negative and destructive and serves only to make us less of a person than we were previously. Fortunately, research in the past 30 years has disclosed much about the nature of pain. The first step toward releasing ourselves from pain involves understanding how pain works.

But Is It All in the Mind?

Pain is not a sense, like touch, sight or hearing. Pain is an emotion. It is the reverse of pleasure, and our language is rich in its imagery. We say, "It pains me to have to tell you," and talk about "the pain of a broken heart" or "painful reality."

People sometimes comment on the pain of others by dismissing it as "psychological," by which they mean imaginary. This is one of many myths about pain, and it stems from a confusion between psychological, or emotional, and imaginary. There is nothing imaginary or unreal about psychological, or emotional, pain.

The fact that you feel pain – for whatever reason – means it is real, so real that if you suffer chronic pain, little else seems to matter.

Pain Gates

Inside our bodies, pain follows a complex pathway from the source of the damage, or disease, to our brain. If, for instance, you drop a six-pack of beer on your big toe, pain messages instantly travel from the site of the injury up the nervous system. On their way to the brain they pass through tiny relay stations at specific points. It is like calling a friend in Toronto from New York City. You pick up the phone in your home and send messages that pass through a telephone exchange in New York. The exchange then transmits them to another relay in Toronto, which in turn sends them to your friend's home. The clarity and sharpness of the messages depend on how the exchanges receive them and pass them on.

Similarly, there are two important relays in our nervous system, which play a vital role in the intensity of pain we suffer. The pain message leaves our big toe and reaches the first relay station, situated in the spinal cord. There, it crosses over the midline of the spine and moves along another pain fiber – up

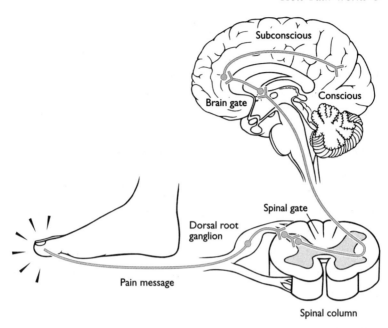

the other side of the body – until it reaches the second relay in the subconscious brain. (These relays are also known as *pain gates*.) The pain message is then passed from there to the conscious brain, which evaluates the warning and reacts immediately. The conscious brain figures, "There's a message coming in from the big-toe nerve. There must be damage down there. Sound the alarm." A millisecond later, we double up in pain and yell "Ouch!"

No Brain – No Pain

The important thing about this is that the pain is experienced with the brain. When an anesthetist puts you to sleep, he or she neutralizes the part of the brain that has the ability to feel pain. While the surgeon then cuts through the skin and removes, say, a lump, and stimulates pain fibers in the process, the part of your body that receives the pain is inactive and cannot feel it. The damage to the tissues is being done, the pain is being produced, but it has nowhere to register.

The brain has to tell us where the pain is coming from. It manages this by learning, over a period of time, which nerves come back from particular areas of the body. The brain of a newborn baby is too immature to localize pain. If you stick a pin into a newborn baby, it rolls into a ball and screams. The baby is aware that something nasty has happened, but does not know where, so it pulls in all four limbs and assumes a protective posture. By the time the baby is one year old, if a pin is stuck into its left leg the left leg moves and the baby screams. It is now aware that the pain has originated from a specific area.

The pain area of the brain works like a telephone switchboard marked out in tiny lights with numbers on them. When the pain bell rings, the brain looks to see which light is flashing and what its number is. Number 123, for instance, might indicate that the pain is coming from the big toe.

This explanation is deceptively simple, because no matter where the big-toe nerve is stimulated along its six-foot (1.8 m) pathway from foot to brain, we will register, and feel, a pain in the big toe. Thus, if the big-toe nerve is stimulated, say, behind the knee because it is pinched in some way, we get a pain down to our big toe. If the sciatic nerve is hit by a nurse's needle, we experience a pain shooting down the leg and into the big toe. If a slipped disk presses on the nerve root that runs back from the big toe, then, accordingly, we feel pain in the big toe.

This is well-known to doctors. If you go to your family physician complaining of severe pain shooting down the back of your leg into your big toe, which came on when you lifted something, it is unlikely that he or she will do a thorough examination of your foot and toe and declare that nothing is wrong because your toe seems all right. The doctor will probably recognize the cause as likely a slipped disk and examine your back first. This kind of *referred pain* is no longer a mystery. Even stimulation of the pathway in the brain will produce pain that appears to come from the beginning of the pathway.

Curiously, the brain does not have pain fibers of its own. The only pain fibers running through the brain come from other parts of the body. They run into specific sites, like highways converging, and so a neurosurgeon can operate directly on the brain without causing pain. There are now special neurosurgical techniques that involve using local anesthetics to numb the tissues and prepare a way into the brain. Probes can then be inserted accurately to locate one specific part of the brain. Once this has been done, an abnormally functioning part of the brain can be treated.

Phantom-Limb Pain

In probing the brain, the surgeon may just touch the pain track, which will produce an experience of pain, again perhaps going down the leg to the big toe if that particular branch of nerves is stimulated. This pain is very real and also located in a specific area of the body, but the message that there is damage there is incorrect.

This explains what is known as *phantom-limb pain*. If people have, for example, a leg amputated, they may have lost 24 inches (about 60 cm) of their body, but the remainder of the nerve that used to come from the amputated area still goes back up to the brain to represent that part of the body. Should that nerve become irritable at the time of the operation or afterward – especially if it has been firing a lot before the operation – then they may experience a phantom limb and feel that the leg is still there.

Often, this is a painful sensation. In fact, some authorities estimate that more than half the people who have a leg amputated suffer phantom-limb pain. Originally, people who had this condition tended not to talk about it. This is perhaps because many were soldiers wounded in battle. Admitting to feeling pain in a limb that had been removed was embarrassing and made others think that something might be mentally wrong with them.

Gradually, amputees began to discuss it with one another and, realizing that the condition was widespread, were able to bring it to the attention of doctors. Although it was known for a long time that the phenomenon occurred, no one really understood why until the development of pain research in the 1960s.

Referred pain can often manifest itself in a heart attack, masquerading as severe pain in the arms, particularly the left arm. Someone arriving at a hospital emergency room complaining of a severe pain in the left arm, looking pale and experiencing slight shock, would be suspected of having a heart attack, even though it is quite clear that the heart is not in their arm! The nerve supply from the heart and the nerves from the arm come from the same group of cells in the embryo. Because as newborns we generally never experience cardiac pain in the learning process, as adults we cannot always identify the pain from heart damage inside the chest. In a similar way, pain from the gall bladder is sometimes experienced behind the right shoulder, rather than in the stomach, below the liver.

The importance of this is that when we say we have a pain and feel it in a specific part of the body, we may be right in that we have pain, but we may be very wrong in exactly where the problem lies. Pain often originates from a specific cause, but once the pain pathway has been open and operating for months or years, other factors come into play. Changes occur within the whole pain transmission process – circuits become hypersensitive and pain messages continue without the original stimulus.

This is the situation many chronic-pain sufferers find themselves in. Their original injury may be clearly understandable and would be expected to cause pain. Perhaps it was a torn muscle or ligament, nerve damage or a broken bone. Ten years later, the original cause has often settled down but the pain continues. The patient, of course, feels that the pain is still coming from one specific part of the body, but when the doctor examines this area nothing wrong can be found. This can lead to misunderstanding between doctor and patient.

Two-Way Traffic

Like the telephone call mentioned earlier, pain messages are two-way traffic. Just as your friend in Toronto reacts to what you say in New York, the brain responds by sending messages back again. Descending pain pathways reach from the conscious brain down to the gates in the subconscious brain and the spinal cord.

The reason for this is that gates are places where the flow of pain messages can be controlled or influenced. By sending responses back, the brain can order the release of chemicals that actually reduce or inhibit pain sensations. These important pain-blocking chemicals, which we manufacture within our bodies, are called *endorphins*. They are the key to controlling pain, and with practice and patience some people can learn how to release them at will. Endorphins – the body's own painkillers – are a powerful, natural weapon for reducing pain.

If we were exposed to the full flow of pain at the time, we would be unable to function properly. In stress or danger, endorphins can block pain to give us time to escape and reach safety – an inbuilt ancient mechanism to ensure survival.

Research has shown that, as individuals, we seem to produce varying amounts of endorphins. Depending on how many we have in our system at any given time, they have a capacity to

The importance of endorphins

If you have a head for mathematics, endorphins work something like this: 1,000 pain messages may start out from an injured toe on their way to the brain. If endorphins block 90 percent of them, only 100 messages may get through the spinal-cord gate. Of those, perhaps only 10 will make it through to the conscious brain. In simple terms, the six-pack of beer you dropped on your foot generated 1,000 "Ouches" of pain, but your brain registered only 10 of them.

On another day, if the gates were only 50 percent effective and you had the bad luck to drop another six-pack on the other foot, something different would happen. If the relays were working at only half capacity, 500 pain messages would pass up the spine, and of those maybe 250 would reach the brain – that's 25 times worse than the previous accident.

In effect you would have felt 25 times more pain, while suffering an identical injury to your toe. This tells us that the severity of what we feel is, in fact, unrelated to the amount of tissue damage we may have suffered, and has much more to do with the state of activity of the nervous system.

block pain a little or a lot. Although endorphins are only one of the factors that influence the pain gates, they are extremely important.

Pain Thresholds and Pain Tolerance

When people with chronic, long-term pain feel depressed or despairing, or they are simply not coping too well, their relay station gates open more than usual, allowing more pain messages through. Even though their original illness or injury does not worsen and the initial number of signals is constant, the pain itself increases. This also happens with many of the other psychological factors that influence pain. This interesting discovery debunked the popular myth of varying *pain thresholds*.

People watching a boxer in the ring may wonder how he has the capacity to take heavy punches. "He doesn't seem to feel them," they say. "He must have a high pain threshold." We all, in fact, have more or less the same pain threshold. When people are asked to hold a metal rod in a laboratory and it is then slowly heated or frozen until they feel discomfort, researchers can almost predict what those cutoff temperatures will be (105°F/43°C for heat and −22° F/−6°C for cold).

What varies from person to person is *pain tolerance*. If we took the same people and asked them to bear as much pain as they possibly could, figures would differ enormously because our personal approach to pain is very important.

When the metal rod experiment was conducted with medical students, they were told that they were going to be subjected to terrible temperatures that could cause tissue damage. The students grimaced in pain and dropped the rods, but in truth the machine was not even connected at the time. The very expectation of pain can be painful.

Pain tolerance not only differs from person to person, but varies within the same person, according to circumstances and the way he or she feels. Experiments show, for instance, that volunteers are prepared to tolerate more pain if friends or colleagues are watching, or even if a reward is offered. Many different factors regulate how much pain we can stand. An entertaining example is the Japanese game show where only contestants who tolerate extremes of pain and embarrassment advance to the next round and win a prize. Some fail miserably, while others show amazing ability in controlling their discomfort.

The difference between pain threshold, which we all share, and pain tolerance, which is different for each individual, is important, because each relates to a quite different type of pain. When we trap a finger in a door, we go beyond our pain threshold – but the pain passes. When we dislocate a shoulder we pass our pain tolerance – but pain becomes intolerable and we consult a doctor.

Fast Pain and Slow Pain

There are two types of pain – *fast* and *slow*. The first triggers a fast-pain message; the second produces a slow, aching sensation. The distinction is clear if you suddenly injure your toe. The first sensation is a sharp flash of pain exactly at the point of contact. This gives way to a burning ache in the general area surrounding the injury. Because messages of fast and slow pain are quite different, they are carried from toe to brain along different kinds of pain pathways.

Fast pain – linked to our pain threshold – warns of sudden localized injury, so that you can pull your foot away, for example. Slow pain, which is sometimes called deep pain, triggers a different reaction. Instead of jerking your body back in a reflex movement, your muscles often go rigid or contract, as though enforcing rest until your body can bring its natural healing into play.

The purpose of fast pain is to attract our attention – to give a sharp warning that we have been damaged in some way that requires a response to avoid further injury. Slow pain is a more complex emotional process, and draws on many kinds of information: memories of similar situations, how members of the family may have reacted in similar circumstances, our anxieties that what we are feeling may lead to something worse.

Slow pain is linked to our pain tolerance, which changes according to our past experience and our present state of mind. Our mental attitude can go a long way toward influencing precisely how much slow pain we feel. Although these pains are very different, both can be helped by distraction: from the simple tactic of a mother rubbing her baby better when he has fallen over, to using hypnosis or music at the dentist's to direct thoughts away from incoming pain messages.

Both fast and slow pain messages are transmitted to the brain by pain *receptors* – a network of tiny nerve endings

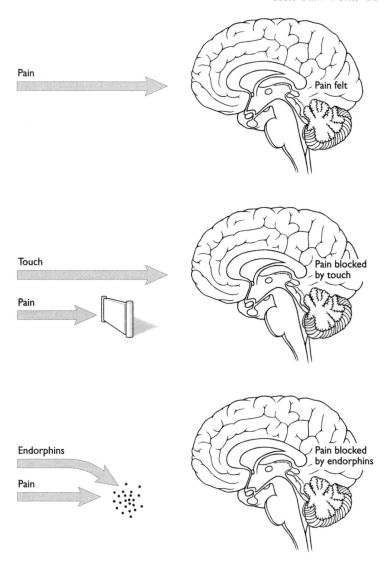

throughout the body that constantly monitor any sensations that might be out of the ordinary.

Fast-pain receptors – *receivers* would be another term for them – lie beneath the surface of the skin. Receptors for slow, or deep, pain share the same locations, but also carry messages from the joints and all the large internal organs of the body. These tiny sense organs pick up a variety of information to send to the brain: whether something is hot or cold to the touch; whether something sharp or blunt is pressing against the skin. Some constantly feed back general information; others report damage or injury. Different receptors transmit differ ent sensations, so, for example, we can distinguish between the prick of a needle and a burn from a hot kettle.

Researchers have discovered that each type of pain recep- tor has its own pathway to carry messages to the brain. Painkillers affect the two types of pain receptors differently. Morphine, for instance, can be used to block the slow mes- sages of chronic pain, but has little effect on the fast-pain mes-

Morphine – key to the discovery of endorphins

Curiously, it was research into the painkilling properties of morphine that led to the discovery of endorphins. Morphine, derived from poppies, is probably the world's oldest painkiller – its use is shown by Egyptian hieroglyphics – but until the early 1970s, no one really understood how it worked. Morphine was found to enter the central nervous system and block the receptors of certain cells – like a key fitting a lock – to cut off pain.

What puzzled researchers was why the body had a lock custom- made to fit the morphine key, when the chances of the average person taking a drug derived from poppies was extremely slim. It soon became clear that the body must have its own painkillers, similar in molecular structure to morphine. The search for them ended in 1975 with the important discovery of endorphins.

This breakthrough led to an explosion of interest in pain research. One result was that compounds have since been discovered in the body that can stimulate the growth of damaged nerves. Morphine has been found to break down into various compounds in the liver. One of them, Morphine 6G, is probably 10 times more potent than morphine itself, and ways in which we process it are currently being investigated.

There are still many exciting discoveries to be made about the body and its capacity for healing itself and overcoming pain.

sages caused by pricking your finger. Painkillers, in other words, work on our pain tolerance, but have little or no effect on our pain threshold.

The body allows us to cope with slow, chronic pain by using pain blockers such as morphine, or our own self-produced endorphins. It also has a way of dealing with fast, reflex pain. When we supply stimulation – for example, we rub a knocked elbow – the number of pain messages transmitted is cut down. The technique has been fine-tuned by medical science, and doctors can achieve the same effect by electrical nerve stimulation, known as TENS, which is described in Chapter 8. Vibration can also have similar benefits.

In simple terms, pain messages open the gates so the messages can flood the brain; the action of rubbing closes the gates and cuts down the number of messages.

In recent years scientists have found that messages are carried along pain pathways as an electrical current. One end of each cell has a receiver, which picks up the pain message, and the other end has a transmitter, a chemical substance, which passes on the pain message when it is released from one nerve ending and spreads to stimulate the next. Some painkilling drugs are designed to act on these *neurotransmitters* and cut down the messages passing down the chain of cells.

Pain Is a Product of Several Factors
Pain is not an illusion, but it is never quite what it seems. Research shows that *nociceptors* are nerve cells that transmit unpleasant impulses to the brain. The word, related to "noxious," refers to the number of pain nerve endings that are stimulated when an injury occurs. Nociception, the transmission of pain impulses along various nerve-fiber pathways to the brain, is not the same thing as pain itself. Along the way, embryo pain messages travel through the gates, or relay sta-

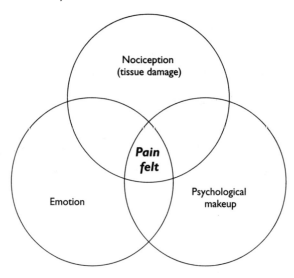

tions, we encountered earlier. Depending upon what is happening at these gates, messages become modified before finally emerging in the brain as a pain warning. Pain, then, is a product of nociception, plus what is happening within the body and to our emotions at a given time.

Because pain tolerance varies according to emotional circumstances, a wounded soldier may feel less pain than someone run over by a bus. The soldier, who perhaps expected to be killed on the battlefield, would be delighted to find himself alive and relieved that he could feel anything at all. The unfortunate pedestrian probably expected to spend a pleasant afternoon without suffering any injuries at all. Their expectations were completely different, and thus their pain is not comparable.

Learn to Control Pain and You'll Overcome It

Pain tolerance is about the amount of pain we expect to receive and are prepared to put up with, depending upon how positive our outlook is.

Here, we have arrived at the central idea of this book: *over-*

coming pain is a matter of learning how to control it. Anyone who suffers chronic pain knows that being in charge of your own pain requires effort, energy and a positive outlook. It is far from easy to achieve because these are the very reservoirs of daily life that pain drains away. However, you can take control by learning how to manage yourself and by understanding what happens when pain takes over.

The Metal Rod Experiment Revisited

Volunteers who take part in pain tolerance experiments are a good illustration of typical reactions to pain. Their responses provide an interesting mirror to hold up to yourself when you suffer pain. The volunteers each have a temperature probe attached to one of their big toes. Connected to the probe is a hand-held button that reverses the temperature as soon as it is pressed. If, for example, the toe becomes hot to a point that they cannot stand, they press the button and the temperature falls until a degree of freezing is reached that is equally uncomfortable.

When they press the button again, the temperature rises through the comfort zone to reach the next high, and so on. As mentioned earlier, most volunteers press the button at around 105°F (43°C) for heat and −22°F (−6°C) for cold.

On a different day, perhaps if some relaxing music is played, their tolerance goes up. There are other influences: if the test controller offers them money to tolerate another degree of temperature, an element of gain is introduced. Most volunteers agree to give it a try, not because we each have our price but, more important, because every pain has its price.

If the volunteer happens to be male and a female test controller asks him if he can stand a few degrees more, the male pride lurking within will inevitably push him to agree. On the other hand, if both volunteer and tester are men, the tester may offer his subject an excuse for trying to be brave. "You don't have to do this," he says. "I couldn't stand that much pain myself." Once the volunteer has this assurance, he usually seizes the opportunity to duck out of the extra pain without losing face.

The button is important because it gives the volunteers control over the pain they experience. In daily life, we are all equipped with similar, personal buttons. The problem is that chronic pain pushes us so far out of control that we forget to use them.

On occasion, testers have secretly disconnected the button to see the reactions of the volunteers. When this vital control is removed, the temperature rises to the pain tolerance level and continues beyond it. The volunteers press the button but, to their alarm, nothing happens. They jump up yelling, as anyone would in the circumstances, and pull the probes from their toes. They have not injured themselves (testers are not in the torture business), but the pain has been sharp enough for them not to entirely trust the experiment controllers again.

When the testers apologize and explain that wiring worked loose, reassuring the volunteers that it is securely plugged in again, human nature takes a hand. The experiment resumes, but this time the volunteers press the button to signal their tolerance level a good few degrees before they actually attain it. As soon as the heat sensation becomes even slightly uncomfortable, they immediately reverse the temperature.

Feeling in Control Is Crucial

There is an interesting lesson about ourselves contained here. The situation is similar to one most of us have experienced in the dentist's chair. You sit down and open your mouth, knowing that the dentist is going to stick instruments into it and probe around. You know that the dentist's next move will be to produce an enormous drill, which you don't like the idea of at all. At the first whine of the drill you stiffen in the chair, and when the dentist hits the tooth nerve, you may hit the roof.

The thought of being unable to tolerate pain has become a self-fulfilling prophecy. You suspected that your dental treatment was going to be unpleasant, and it was. In reality, half the problem lay in your apprehension, your lack of control and, finally, your embarrassment at screaming in front of the dentist and his assistant. Your state of mind allowed many more messages than necessary through the pain gate.

The scenario, however, need not have proceeded like that. An understanding dentist might have said, "Hold up your hand the moment you feel any pain. When that happens, I'll stop immediately. You won't feel any pain longer than a split second."

You would have sat in the chair more relaxed and reassured. Although the dentist might have been doing something that felt uncomfortable, you would have known you had control over it. The difference is that you could go right up to your tolerance level and stand the pain for several minutes, simply because of this control. This concept is important: how much pain you are prepared to tolerate depends upon the degree of control you have over it. You can learn how to control pain by being able to tolerate more of it, so that the pain in turn becomes less unpleasant.

Many people in chronic pain find themselves out of control and desperately seek someone else to fix their pain for them. Their *locus of control* is poor. The more doctors they visit, the more hopeless and inadequate they feel as patients. Eventually, they may find themselves at a pain clinic, where the first daunting words they hear may not be quite what they expected: "We are not going to fix the pain for you, but we can teach you how to cope with it yourself."

At this point, some people lose interest before they have begun. They want to continue their search for the mythical "right" doctor who will magically take away their pain for them. In the course of their quest, which may last a lifetime, they may encounter doctors who offer to operate, prescribe new drugs for them, possibly even hit them on the head with a silver hammer if they are prepared to pay the fee.

They have channeled all their valuable energy into searching for someone to cure them, instead of using that energy to help themselves. Because they have a poor, or external, locus of control, they are not interested in making an effort to cope without someone else offering to carry the burden. In effect, it becomes the sufferer's equivalent of the search by the knights of the Round Table for the Holy Grail – a noble and understandable quest, but doomed to absolute failure because the Holy Grail did not exist.

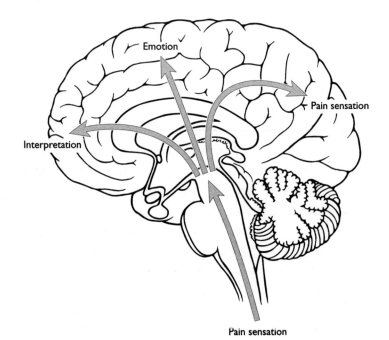

The purpose of a pain management program, and this book, is to help you recenter that lost locus of control and work on being in control again. The results can be tremendously encouraging, both physically and mentally, and in terms of restored confidence. The program also aims to help stimulate a positive outlook, which is essential not only for overcoming pain but for rebuilding a normal lifestyle.

Help Yourself By Thinking Positively

A great step toward doing the things you used to do is achieved through positive thinking – not a fanciful notion confined to "how to improve yourself" books, but an important technique for training the mind to influence the body.

This is clearly illustrated in ulcer pain. Joe, a regional sales manager for a brewery, was a typical patient. He had lost considerable time from work while being treated for a peptic ulcer. After treatment, he was free from pain for six months and was about to go on holiday.

To clear a backlog of paperwork before his break, Joe had been burning the midnight oil, and he was suddenly struck by severe indigestion. His *emotional* reaction was one of panic. The only thought in Joe's mind was that his ulcer had flared again and another depressing period of illness loomed on the horizon. This was followed immediately by his *interpretational* reaction: "My ulcer's back. My holiday will have to be canceled. Everything is ruined."

Together, the two reactions caused so much stress that his stomach released excessive acid, which, naturally, made the ulcer much worse. In short, another self-fulfilling prophecy. By allowing his emotions to become worked up and by visualizing a series of doom-laden events Joe, in effect, made them a reality. Psychologists call this *catastrophizing*, which is a perfect description. In a similar way, stress caused by negative thinking and catastrophizing by someone who has back pain can precipitate a muscle spasm that makes his or her whole condition worse.

Logically, Joe need not have put himself through such double despair. If he had had a stronger locus of control, he might have adopted a more positive approach to his ulcer — perhaps taking antacids, stopping smoking, adjusting his drinking habits and making a point of putting time aside each day to relax. His stomach would have secreted less acid, and by the time his holiday came around, the ulcer would probably have been well on the way to healing completely. Rather than miss his break, he could have returned home feeling refreshed and probably quite smug at his achievement.

Positive self-help, which would have resulted in a completely different pain scenario, requires more energy, effort, discipline and dedication. In the end, however, it pays off. Acquiring the habit of positive thinking, which we shall look at in depth later, also involves learning how to trick the body into drawing upon its own healing resources.

A similar approach was used by estate agent Tom, who suffered from high blood pressure but learned a form of relaxation to cope with the stress of city driving. If he was plowing through heavy traffic, late for an appointment, the sight of a red traffic light was almost like pulling a lever that sent his blood pressure soaring.

A positive approach made the red light trigger a completely different response. Tom would be delighted to have a whole minute in which to relax completely. The red light presented a wonderful opportunity to take time out from the hurly-burly of city driving and lower his stress level. By the time the light changed to green, he felt good, less anxious, and fresh for his appointment. Unlike the harassed drivers behind him, the more traffic lights he encountered, the happier he became.

This positive approach has been demonstrated to be highly effective in lowering blood pressure. The problem is that when our physical and mental resources are low, summoning the effort to look after the body is very demanding. It seems easier to reach for a painkiller.

But placing the problem of pain in someone else's hands is not really the easiest method at all. Joe's stomach ulcer and Tom's high blood pressure are symptoms of other things happening in life that usually result in stress. Like pain, they cannot be swept under the carpet by constantly relying on medication. When pills are used to suppress symptoms, stress – like water forced through a leaky joint – will inevitably emerge in other ways, until you find yourself on the familiar treadmill again.

Employing positive attitudes for the ulcer or relaxation for blood pressure makes you healthier in every sense – not just physically and mentally, but by preventing further problems that might arise. When you succumb to reaching for a pill every time you feel ill, you never address the real issues that need to be resolved. The pill may mask the symptoms, but beneath the illusion you are still sick. The real solution lies on the reverse of the coin – in a realization that your emotional and mental outlook can greatly affect the way you cope with pain.

TWO

Painkiller – or Bitter Pill?

Few people manage to go through life without turning for help to painkillers. Chronic-pain sufferers often take them in quantity, and it is easy to understand why. As pain becomes more difficult to cope with, reaching for medication to get through the day becomes an instinctive reaction.

It has been said that most of us suffer at least one twinge of pain a day for reasons that are never discovered. Judging by the vast range of remedies on drugstore shelves, anyone would be forgiven for thinking that most people are in pain all the time. Painkillers are now so commonplace that we take them without thinking. But just as we need to understand why we are in pain and how pain works, it is equally important to know something about the pills we take. Are they doing their job? Are they the right pills for your particular condition? How long should you take them for? Indeed, should you be taking them at all?

The Analgesic Ladder
The longer you have chronic pain, the more stubbornly it

refuses to go away and, in turn, forces you to search for stronger medications to control it. Drug treatment for pain is referred to by doctors and pharmacists as the *analgesic ladder*. Most painkillers fall into three groups: acetylsalicylic acid, or ASA (aspirin); codeine; or morphine. Chronic-pain patients are progressed up the ladder by their physicians when the pain worsens and they can find no other relief.

If you have pain at this moment and are using off-the-shelf remedies or drugs prescribed by your doctor, they will probably be medications on one of the three rungs of the analgesic ladder (see drug table at end of book).

Off-the-shelf drugs are usually rung one, or aspirinlike; codeine and morphine, rungs two and three, are controlled substances (i.e., need a doctor's prescription) because they can be abused. (Some off-the-shelf remedies have a slight amount of codeine in them.) Fortunately, drugs recommended by your doctor are usually in the first or second category. In general, morphinelike drugs are not used for chronic pain. However, they may be used in special cases.

Patients who move up the ladder seeking relief find that some drugs have greater or less effect on their pain and, in doing so, make physical and mental demands of them. The initial optimism at embarking on a new course of drug treatment often distracts people from considering the side effects that may follow.

Even the aspirin group, the mildest pills on the lowest rung of the ladder, can have unexpected side effects. Perhaps more than any other type of medication, people take these simple analgesics without any basic understanding of the drugs. The painkillers they buy may be entirely inappropriate for their condition.

This, of course, is not to say that simple painkillers are ineffective or bad for you. Many are the result of sophisticated pharmaceutical research. They have an excellent effect in relieving minor pains that do not require a visit to the doctor. It is a question of tailoring the particular product to your type of pain. Keeping a supply of simple analgesics handy is sensible self-management, but they should be types that you know from experience do not upset you.

We tend to choose a particular brand of simple analgesic from habit, often conditioned by what we were given during childhood or what we are most familiar with. Pharmacy shelves, as we have said, are stacked with analgesics, but none has ever consistently been proved best. Off-the-shelf treatments usually contain aspirin, ibuprofen or acetaminophen. Quite often you find them in combination with other substances, but this does not normally offer any particular advantage.

Nonsteroidal Anti-inflammatory Drugs

The ASA-like group, including aspirin and ibuprofen, are known as *nonsteroidal anti-inflammatory drugs* (NSAIDs). Here is how they work.

Damaged tissues release *prostaglandins,* hormones that irritate nerve endings and help nerve fibers carry pain messages to the brain. Generally, over-the-counter remedies inhibit production of prostaglandins, and so reduce inflammation and pain. NSAIDs are sold by your local pharmacist in smaller doses than those prescribed by your family physician. Recent evidence, however, suggests that some of the side effects of NSAIDS, which include the worsening of even mild cases of kidney disease, can occur even at these lower doses.

ASA, common to most simple analgesics, is sold everywhere. (ASA is called "aspirin" in the U.S.; in Canada, "Aspirin" is a brand name.) ASA and acetaminophen work

Rules of thumb for taking off-the-shelf analgesics safely

- Aside from the obvious precautions of following the instructions and not exceeding the dosage, it is important to read carefully what the medicine contains. Someone allergic to ASA, for example, may need to avoid other off-the-shelf medications that contain ASA-like ingredients, such as magnesium salicylate, choline salicylate and sodium salicylate.
- Unless your physician says otherwise, you should impose a cutoff period of 10 days for over-the-counter painkillers. Children and teenagers should take them for no longer than 5 consecutive days. For all ages, medication should never be taken more than 3 days when there is fever.
- Similarly, don't take ASA in the final 3 months of pregnancy, unless your doctor recommends it, since it can cause bleeding in both mother and child.
- Reye's syndrome is rare but potentially fatal. Children and teenagers should not take ASA for chicken pox, flu or flulike symptoms. No one under 18 should take ASA at all without specific instructions from a doctor.
- Don't take ASA for two weeks before surgery unless your doctor specifically recommends its use.

equally well; they just work by different means and have different side effects.

ASA can usually be taken quite safely, but in some people it may cause nausea, indigestion, dizziness or ringing in the ears. Some people who take this painkiller get bleeding in the gastrointestinal tract, and people admitted to the hospital with severe internal bleeding have often taken it in the previous 24 hours. If you experience any bleeding, asthma, skin rashes or confusion, stop taking ASA immediately and see a doctor.

Unless the circumstances are exceptional, ASA should never be used by people with a history of stomach ulcers, bleeding

Ask your doctor

Because the vast majority of drugs on the analgesic ladder are likely to be prescribed by family physicians, it is important to use your family doctor as effectively as possible. The more you complain about pain, the more likely it is you will be prescribed stronger drugs, so there are questions you should ask:

- Are these pills addictive?
- What side effects do they have?
- Is it advisable to take them long-term?
- Is there a pill I can take less often?

problems, severe indigestion, asthma, liver or kidney disease or severe allergies, or by pregnant women, lactating mothers or children under 18. In the case of young people, evidence suggests that ASA may be a factor in Reye's syndrome, a rare but serious form of liver failure.

Acetaminophen also has side effects. The mildest are skin rashes and allergies and the worst liver or kidney damage, but only in cases of overdose. It is therefore essential *never* to take more than the prescribed dose, particularly since doing so does not produce any extra pain relief.

If you are in any doubt about what type of medication you have been given, ask your doctor or consult the drug list at the back of the book.

Climbing the Analgesic Ladder – the Morphines and Codeines

On the second rung of the analgesic ladder are the codeinelike drugs, and on the third rung the morphinelike drugs. Morphine is an addictive drug, and while it is excellent for acute pain such as postoperative pain or heart attacks and some cases of cancer pain, it is not used for chronic pain, as a general rule. When it is, problems may be minimized by taking the drug regularly, rather than only in response to pain. Addiction is a concern when morphine is used for nonpain reasons such as mood disorders and social problems.

When codeinelike drugs, such as oxycodone and propoxyphene, are given for more than six months, the same problem of addiction can occur. This is why it is especially important to ask your doctor about the possible addictive nature of the drugs, and if it is reasonable to take them long-term.

There are also questions you should ask yourself. If you regularly take drugs for chronic pain, you may understandably want to cut down on them. Are they doing their job? More specifically – can you function normally while taking them?

A lawyer suffered severe pain and regularly took a drug on the codeine rung of the analgesic ladder. He was concerned that it might not be suitable for him. In conversation, it emerged that not only could he work in court without problems, but on weekends he played tennis or went hiking. He was advised to continue with his medication. He functioned normally on his particular drug and clearly would not have been able to cope as well without it.

Other chronic-pain patients taking drugs have painted a different picture when asked about their daily activities. Their medication may be ineffective, resulting in a profoundly negative effect on their physical and mental well-being.

Relying entirely on pills to relieve pain means that any gain you expected may be overshadowed by demands the drugs make.

Secondary Analgesics

Alongside the analgesic ladder are drugs known as *secondary analgesics*. These medications usually have another prime purpose, but doctors have discovered that one of their spinoff effects is to reduce certain types of pain. The most important of these are drugs that affect the central nervous system in some way so as to modify pain. They include tranquilizers, anticonvulsants and antidepressants.

Tranquilizers

Many patients prescribed pills for pain relief don't realize that they may be taking a tranquilizer, such as a benzodiazepine. These include diazepam and lorazepam. There are a variety of common names or brand names for these tranquilizers.

This particular family of secondary analgesics is intended to work as a muscle relaxant, especially in cases of back pain. These drugs too are addictive if taken regularly. Patients preoccupied with chronic pain may not realize that it is unwise to take this group of drugs for longer than six weeks. At the end of that period muscle relaxants should be discontinued; otherwise the medication takes over the function of the muscles. People suffering from, say, back pain caused by muscle spasms may discover that their muscles are unable to relax of their own accord again without the pills. The result is that they no longer have control over their muscle spasm, because the work has been taken over entirely by the pills. They then become locked into a cycle of chronic pain.

It is important that any of the benzodiazepine family of secondary analgesics be regarded as short-term drugs. When they are taken for longer periods, patients become physically and mentally dependent for the temporary sense of relief and euphoria.

Anticonvulsants

Another group of secondary analgesics is the *anticonvulsants*, which are usually used to treat epilepsy. Chronic pain is not normally associated with epilepsy, but the ability of these drugs to stabilize nerve membranes may be the reason they benefit some people. They work on epilepsy by stopping the hyper-irritability that produces messages going down to the muscles to make them twitch. In chronic pain, they work by reducing excessive electrical activity within the brain itself or within the spinal cord, which brings pain messages back up to the brain.

Anticonvulsants have proved particularly useful in providing pain relief for shooting pain or knifelike stabbing pain. These are pains that involve nerve irritation or nerve damage, such as post-shingles neuralgia, diabetic neuropathy or the almost unbearable pain of trigeminal neuralgia. They can be so severe that they completely change the sufferer's personality and lifestyle. Here's a case in point.

Sidney was known as an eccentric recluse. On the few occasions he ventured out, he had an unkempt beard and wore his coat collar pulled high over his head, even on the hottest day. He looked suspicious and deranged and his face was pale and gaunt.

Unknown to his neighbors, Sidney was a victim of extreme pain – in his case trigeminal neuralgia – which makes the face so sensitive that eating, shaving, talking or even exposure to the slightest breeze can cause agony. Sydney rarely ate because it hurt to eat; he seldom talked because talking was painful. He hardly ever went out and had no one to help him. When he arrived at the clinic, he was a lonely, frightened man and a total prisoner of his pain.

He was given anticonvulsant tablets used for treating epilepsy. By his next visit there was a remarkable transformation. For the first time in years his collar was folded down, his manner was more confident and his neuralgic pain was noticeably more under control. Sidney eventually went on to have a simple nerve block operation to complete his treatment and his life changed completely. (Further information on the treatment of trigeminal neuralgia can be found in chapter 8.) The lesson here is that such pills are useful tools of treatment if taken wisely and effectively.

Even so, anticonvulsants may have side effects with long-term use. Patients can become unsteady on their feet and prone to blood disorders. Some may have to take anticonvulsants for years, but with careful monitoring and reduced dosages when necessary, the unpleasant effects of the drug can be controlled. Newer drugs, with fewer side effects, are available.

Antidepressants

Other commonly prescribed secondary analgesics are the antidepressants. They are not addictive and can be used for long periods, particularly for peripheral nerve damage, such as shingles or the "burning foot" sensation of diabetes. They are thought to help by interfering with serotonin and noradrenaline, chemical transmitters of nerve impulses.

They can be used when there is no depression, although mild depression often accompanies chronic pain. Some can have uncomfortable side effects, such as fatigue and bladder-emptying problems, but these are less of a problem with newer drugs.

Some antidepressants have a sedative effect and may be taken only at night. They may help chronic-pain sufferers to sleep restfully. The pain may be just as bad during the day, but a welcome opportunity to sleep helps people cope better.

Secondary analgesics can be an enormous help to patients. Ken, a warehouse worker, struggled to hold down his job while suffering chronic back pain. His family doctor prescribed codeine, which did not help at all. He was then prescribed amitriptyline (an antidepressant), which greatly relieved the problem.

What suited Ken, however, may not be appropriate for the next patient to come along. Response to drugs varies from person to person. It is important to take a balanced view of what your pills are actually doing to help cut down pain. You should not take steps to reduce them simply because you don't like the idea of taking drugs. If they are generally working to reduce pain and allow you to lead a normal life, there is no reason to stop taking them.

Many medications, however, do not have these ideal properties. Drugs on the codeine and morphine rungs of the analgesic ladder, for instance, tend to suppress the body's natural ability to inhibit pain. It is not fully understood why this occurs, but it would not be unreasonable to imagine that drugs such as morphine subjugate the body's own pain-reducing mechanism by inhibiting the production of endorphins.

If we see the body as full of tiny endorphin-producing factories, turning out substances to combat pain, and imagine the "market" suddenly flooded with morphine, this seems natural. When morphine provides pain inhibitors of similar molecular shape, the body's own endorphin factories shut down. When the time comes to reopen, they may be in no fit state to do this and may be unable to produce endorphins. Consequently, the patient will suffer out of all proportion to the disease.

Here are some guidelines to help you decide about pain medication:

• Simple painkillers, providing they help without side effects, are worthwhile.
• Stronger painkillers, providing they allow increased or normal activity, are also acceptable.

- If painkillers are not helping, they should be tapered off, with the advice of your doctor.
- If you feel you have an overreliance, physical or mental, on pain pills, you are probably best stopping them in the long run.

THREE

Regaining Control

One of the many illusions of pain is that the more it increases, the worse our condition becomes. Pain sufferers turn to their doctor, hoping something can be done to relieve their misery by treating the root cause. The more severe the pain becomes, the more desperately they seek help. If the illness can be cured, they argue, then naturally the pain will go away.

Chronic Pain Is a Separate Entity

As patients on pain management programs discover, this is not necessarily so. One of the great revelations about pain is that it should be considered as a completely separate entity from the injury or disease that originally caused it. Realizing this is an important step toward using your own inbuilt coping skills to deal with pain.

The key to long-term pain control lies within you, rather than with a doctor who may prescribe drugs or surgery. If you suffer chronic pain, this is not an easy concept to grasp, because pain has a habit of altering perception, attitude and general outlook. If you can't think straight, it is difficult to put your pain in perspective.

The first step in overcoming this lies in realizing that *the severity of pain is not related to the severity of illness*. Anyone can die just as easily from a painless heart attack as from a painful one. Some forms of cancer, particularly the leukemias, can be quite malignant without being painful at all. Other types of cancer are extremely painful, but this has no bearing on their severity.

Changing your attitude to pain by placing it in perspective has a great effect on how much pain you can tolerate without it interfering with normal daily life.

Hospital emergency room staff, for example, know that some people wheeled in with horrific injuries do not seem to be in much discomfort, while people with minor sprains can be in agony. Similarly, some of those patients with minor sprains causing intense pain may find it has disappeared by the time they reach the emergency room. Others with a sprain may at first feel no pain, yet be crying by the time they arrive at the hospital.

Obviously, there is a principle here worth considering. The injury or illness may be the same, but the pain does not relate to its severity. In other words, *pain is often out of all proportion to disease*.

Pain Tolerance Is Learned

Changing your attitude to pain is not as easy as it may sound. Coping with pain is something we unconsciously learn as children and are conditioned to as we grow up. How we learn to tolerate pain is so deep-rooted that it varies from person to person, family to family, even country to country.

The important point is that within these groups certain

people will cope differently from others. Introverts, extroverts, people who are naturally relaxed and those generally tense all possess traits that regulate how much pain they experience and complain of.

People who suffer physical and sexual abuse as children are more likely to suffer chronic pain than is the general population. If this applies to you, you should seek help from a trained counselor or psychologist, through your doctor.

Once patients begin to talk about themselves, family histories of pain are often uncovered. If, for example, a child has a parent who suffered from chronic pain and could not cope very well with it, there is a strong chance that the child will not learn to cope with pain either. Alternatively, people who had a parent who was ill but rarely made the family aware of it may grow up to be good at coping themselves.

Conditioning of this kind is hard to undo, but you can make progress toward it by trying to put your pain in perspective. Most acute pain warns of tissue damage. When a caveman woke up to find a saber-toothed tiger gnawing his leg, the pain message instantly told him to run as fast as he could. It warned him that he needed an acute reaction to the life-threatening situation he found himself in. His attitude to pain, putting it mildly, would be a major response. Pain would be the most vital thing he was feeling and his brain would rate it as the most important sensation.

This rule does not apply to chronic pain. If someone has had a painfully arthritic knee for years, then the pain, in some ways, is not particularly important anymore. The sufferer can argue with his or her subconscious, "The pain this morning does not mean that there is any new disease in my knee. It was hurting years ago and will probably continue to hurt in the future. I can safely ignore the pain because it is no different from the way it has been before."

Your attitude to pain, therefore, should not be that it is something enormous and terrible because you have suffered so long. By changing your perspective and rationalizing what you feel, you can tell yourself, "If the pain has been there for that length of time, perhaps I don't need to take so much notice of it."

In chronic-pain cases there is rarely any ongoing disease process to worry about, yet patients locked into their pain often fear the opposite. They feel that the longer their pain persists or the worse it becomes, the more their illness is progressing and taking hold of them.

Again, pain and illness are two separate entities. Once you convince yourself of that, you are halfway to changing your attitude toward pain. If your pain happens to be particularly bad today, try to place it in perspective. Some days may be good and others unbearable, but it does not mean that you are more ill and your health is deteriorating.

Understand Your Doctor's Perspective

Occasionally, the situation may be made worse by a physician who feels unable to help a particular patient. A doctor may examine someone's back and say without thinking, "You've got the spine of a 90-year-old." The patient goes home brooding over every word, forgetting that some 90-year-olds live a completely normal life.

The fact is that family doctors and orthopedic surgeons sometimes find themselves challenged by long-term pain sufferers. Patients look to them hopefully for recovery, but in many cases therapeutic treatment is impossible. A surgeon may scrutinize the X-rays, shake his or her head and remark, "Your back is in a terrible state. I'm sorry, but there's nothing I can do for you. It's beyond repair." Doctors, after all, are in the business of making people well. They may feel inadequate dealing with long-term cases where pills have little effect and chances of recovery are slim.

Chronic-pain patients may leave a doctor's office feeling badly treated, but doctors may also have their own problems. When they treat patients, they expect their conditions to improve. If, visit after visit, chronic-pain sufferers fail to respond, doctors may have difficulty coping too. In the back of their minds they see a waiting-room full of patients whom they probably have a reasonable chance of curing.

Subconsciously, they may think that if they can dispense with the "incurable" long-term sufferer and move on to more easily treated cases, they will feel more fulfilled. They may rationalize their frustration by bluntly telling such patients just how bad their condition is, in the hope that these people will go away and try to come to terms with it. That way, no one can blame the doctor for a failure to "cure."

Unfortunately, this negative approach seldom works in practice. While it is true that some people desperately want a diagnosis, once they have been baldly informed of the facts they feel unable to cope. After badgering the doctor to be honest, they mull over the diagnosis and conclude that it would have been better never to know they had an arthritic spine. The prospect of being crippled for life proves to be too much to bear.

If instead the surgeon had commented, "Your back has had more than the average wear and tear. But it's no worse than similar cases I've seen. I certainly don't think you need surgery," then the patient's attitude might have been completely different.

Professional soccer players quite often have damaged knees,

yet still turn out to play every weekend. There is no question that they are in pain, but they do not allow it to affect their performance. People should evaluate their pain – even to the point of obtaining a second opinion – and find out if there is any reason they should not be more mobile.

Obviously, if you have a fractured leg you should not walk on it and make it worse. However, if you have a bad back and indulge in some activity that makes it hurt the next day, this does not mean that you have damaged yourself. It more likely indicates that you are unfit. The way to overcome this is to achieve modest targets until, with practice, you can get around with less discomfort.

The importance of targeting, as we shall see, is never to lower your expectations because of fear of hurting yourself. Occasionally, some patients have had postexercise pain the day after doing their tai chi exercises and have complained to their physician of stiffness and discomfort. The doctor, who understandably had more pressing matters to attend to, advised them to stop exercising if it hurt!

What the patients failed to understand was that, subconsciously, they were engineering a situation that would allow them to stop exercising. If they had asked, more reasonably, "Is it harming me to have this pain?" it is probable that their doctor would have thought not and have advised them to go on. Providing your doctor says it is safe for you to do gentle exercise, you should adopt a positive attitude, believing that it will improve your ability to cope with pain.

Reduce Your Pain with the Right Attitude

Chronic pain changes our attitude. It forces us to forget that we were once positive people and, like water, to always seek the lowest level: to err on the side of caution and compromise, to constantly seek out the negative, until we become less of a person than we were before.

This need not be so. Experience shows that people who determinedly work to change their attitude, and make a positive effort to do more, discover that their tolerance to pain improves. Here is Barbara's experience after suffering chronic back pain from a car accident: "After the usual merry-go-round of family physician, hospital, specialist, family physician, hospital, painkiller, operations and injections, I was bluntly told that nothing could be done for my injury and pain. I felt very angry. I had lost my job, my hobbies, my social life. I was at war with the world and my family.

"I could hardly do a thing for myself, the pain in my back was so bad. I was also very stiff – all my back muscles were in spasm and I had no control over them. Through this period my family physician, family and friends were very supportive. They stopped me from going into deep depression.

"I am not a loser and would not accept the fact that this situation was to be my life. I was 42 years old and had no intention of going through life pill-popping. I didn't care what it took – I was determined to have myself a normal life again. When my doctor suggested a pain clinic, I was ready to try anything.

"At my appointment, I was told that I must be prepared for four weeks' hard work, and that would be just the tip of the iceberg. The doctor said he could not cure my pain, but he could give me a better quality of life. I was desperate. I was prepared to try anything and give it 101 percent. Deep inside I was scared and very apprehensive and fearful of doing myself more damage.

"I attended the clinic not knowing what to expect and was

introduced to the team and the program. Everyone was so helpful, so understanding. People cared. Everyone wanted me to do well and nothing was too much trouble. Even the other people on the course, who were in pain themselves, encouraged me. I felt that there was light at the end of the tunnel. At last I was coming out of the labyrinth of darkness.

"I found the exercises very painful and at one time I thought I was going to die, but I worked even harder. The relaxation helped me find a way through the pain and my negative thoughts. At last, my body was doing what I wanted it to do, not what the pain wanted. Once I realized that hurt did not mean harm, I really pushed myself.

"I began to realize that self-discipline and self-control were a necessity. Slowly, the fear and the anger started to fade. These two emotions would pull me back if I didn't let go. I learned not just to rest, but to relax.

"Family and friends have seen a difference in me. I am starting to laugh and joke again. The quality of my life has improved. I have started my keep-fit lessons again and I am now walking my dog. Generally, I am doing much more for myself and relying less on others. I still have pain, but with discipline and self-control, I rule my body and mind.

"I will not let the pain take over. Today, I take fewer painkillers and hope to decrease them even more.

"At home, I am trying to forget the negative life I lived for three years. I am now positive again, in complete control. You can be in pain and enjoy life. With hard work and dedication, pain can be controlled without losing any of the quality of life."

Barbara changed her life by developing a positive attitude and putting her pain in perspective.

You Can Do More Than You Think

Many chronic-pain sufferers do not go dancing or bowling because they believe that the pain they may suffer next day indicates they have done themselves damage. They will hurt, but only because they have not been active for so long. It is important to learn the difference between damage pain and postexercise pain. If people last danced 15 years ago, they cannot possibly know if they cannot dance today. It may be difficult and something of an ordeal, but what they are really saying is that they *won't* dance. They have made a judgment that is backed by fear, not fact. Their decision is that they simply will not be able to do it again.

What they should do is *un*decide and tell themselves, "I'd like to dance again. It's not going to be easy, but I'll try to see if I can work up to it."

What we have here is another of pain's illusions. Pain encourages you to play safe so that it, not you, remains in control. Remember, *hurt does not mean harm.* Chronic-pain sufferers have a potential far greater than they imagine.

Having the right attitude to pain brings us back to locus of control – regaining control over yourself and the pain in your body. If you give up at the first twinge, then pain is running you.

People beginning pain programs have an external locus of control, by which we mean that they expect other people to do things for them to help their pain. As soon as they are in pain, they stop their activities and allow the pain to come through and dominate their lives. Learning to change your attitude means getting on with things and depressing the amount of pain that comes through for the length of a given activity. It means closing your pain gates and telling yourself that nothing will stop you from going on with a particular exercise.

The prospect of a reward can help you

Fakirs who lie on beds of nails or fire walkers who stroll over hot coals all withstand a certain amount of pain to achieve a goal. Beds of nails, for example, are made to precise specifications in which the nails are grouped closely to reduce the pain. If there were only half a dozen nails on the board, not even the most experienced fakir could tolerate the pain.

The trick lies in reducing the amount of pain they allow through and coping with it. Such performers know they are not going to physically harm themselves because they have done it many times before, and have often seen their fathers and grandfathers do the same.

What also helps them reduce the pain to an acceptable level is the reward at the end – it may be money, kudos, mental satisfaction or some kind of mystical experience. The fakirs still hurt, but the payback enables them to allow only a certain amount of pain through, which they can adequately cope with.

Learning to Close Your Pain Gates

Learning to control your pain gates is like learning to wiggle your ears. We all obviously have innate abilities – raising a leg or moving our toes. Other abilities, such as being able to twitch our ears, are more hidden. We all have a muscle behind each ear and a nerve running from it to the brain. So, in theory, we should all be able to wiggle our ears. However, not everyone knows how to do it in practice. Perhaps an average of one person in ten can perform this trick, but if you ask these people to teach the other nine, they do not know where to begin. They have no idea *how* they do it, only that they can. The others agree that it is possible in theory, but somehow they can't.

In a similar way, the same ten people could close their pain gates and block a great proportion of their pain. They understand how it is possible to do it – that they all possess the mechanism to make it happen – but perhaps only one of them is able to put it into practice. As in juggling three balls, there is a difference between admiring someone's ability and acquiring the knack yourself.

When a thousand pain specialists attended an international conference in Florence, Italy, they broke after one of the sessions and wandered into the square outside the conference hall. A crowd was gathered around a man walking barefoot over broken glass and then holding his feet in a candle flame. The pain doctors gathered around, fascinated, and asked if he felt anything.

The performer claimed he felt no pain at all. Then one of the Italian pain specialists gave him some money and he talked more frankly about how he earned his living. He admitted that the glass and the candle flame were quite painful, but he was able to suppress the pain because of the money he stood to collect at the end of each performance. No one in the crowd, or indeed any of the doctors, could have withstood so much pain, but the performer was able to modify the pain because of that secondary gain.

When we consider pain gates, it is important to remember that those who can't close them are the ones who allow their lives to revolve entirely around the fact that they are ill and in pain. Their frustration begins when they discover that it is possible to close pain gates and have less pain. They try, but nothing happens because their subconscious – which is always logical about such things – prevents them. "Just a minute," their subconscious insists. "Your pain is important to you. You seem to need your pain gates open to allow as much pain through as possible to tell you something is wrong."

So the subconscious, quite rightly, reasons this way: "You are asking me to close the gates and cut down pain, but I can't really believe you mean what you say. As soon as I open the gates and allow the pain through, you stop what you are doing and take a pill. This tells me that pain is the most important thing in your life. You give it your full attention whenever it demands it. If you really didn't want to know about pain, you wouldn't take any notice."

The subconscious is never going to learn to close the gates because the sufferers confirm they are ill by stopping whatever they are doing every time pain messages pass through.

Set Targets and Don't Give Up
The only way to effectively convince your subconscious is not to make promises, but to *live* in such a way that it believes you mean business. This means not grinding to a halt and giving up every time you feel a twinge. It means setting yourself a target for a particular activity and accomplishing it, whether the pain comes through or not.

If, for example, you have decided to pedal an exercise bike for 10 minutes or to take a 10-minute walk, it does not matter that you feel pain after six or eight minutes; you still have to go the distance and complete the 10 minutes. If you have been assured medically that this cannot harm you, there is no reason to give in to pain anymore.

Admitting defeat is not the easy way out. The sooner you give up before reaching your target, the greater the chances that you will feel more pain, not less, because you are giving your subconscious the approval to let pain through. You have not convinced it that you really mean what you say. Cave in early and your subconscious will argue, "I knew you were going to feel pain after six minutes, so next time I will open the gates after five minutes to warn you not to push yourself too far."

Given the opportunity, your subconscious becomes one of those annoying people who think they know best and try to organize your life for you. Sometimes, you just have to be insistent, to put your foot down and prove that you are in charge. Otherwise, on the next occasion, your subconscious will decide to open the gates after four minutes to play safe, and so on. The more easily you give up, the more painful it becomes, and any progress you had hoped to make vanishes.

Once you've decided on your target, it becomes vitally important to stick to it. You may find that the activity is easier than you thought and you feel you can go on for 12 minutes. This is almost as bad as giving up early, because you are cheating your subconscious.

You have to prove that, when you say something, you mean

Three self-help success stories

Ellen, 54, was in so much pain that she could not stand the touch of clothes on her back. Eventually, she joined a pain management program. "Instead of feeling alone, frightened and suicidal, I was shown various methods of self-help and was amazed at the difference they made to my life. I still have chronic pain every single day, but rather than dwell on all the things I once enjoyed doing, I find other ways around it. For instance, I gave up typing because of the pain in my hands from arthritis. By setting myself targets, I bought myself an electric typewriter and was thrilled when people asked me to type for them. I have now enrolled for a course in word processing so that I can extend my interests."

Terry, a bus driver, suffers from chronic back pain: "For years, I avoided using my left hand and arm because I thought I would automatically give myself more pain. This has been proved incorrect. My plans now are to continue with exercises, as I didn't realize how unfit I was until I started doing them. I have just begun to go swimming again – a marvelous exercise and one that I had simply got out of the habit of doing."

Kay suffered chest pains following a pulmonary embolism: "I felt desperate. Desperate at the way in which fear of pain was taking my life over. I had stopped exercising a long time ago in case I made the pain worse. I avoided making social engagements for fear of not being well enough to go. In the end, friends became fed up with me canceling dates. Understanding the psychology of pain has really helped me. I realize how protective of my body I had become and I am thankful I am now through the barrier. I am less fearful and analytical of my pain because I know I have the tools to cope with it."

it. If you make a deal for 10 minutes and exceed it, your subconscious becomes confused. It prepared itself to keep the gates closed for 10 minutes because it knew you were determined to stick to your decision. As soon as you increased the time, it believed you were no longer in control and felt it might as well open the gates at 3 minutes as at 12.

Setting targets means

- thinking through what you intend to do;
- taking complete control of yourself;
- having the right attitude;
- sticking to what you say.

It does not mean vague, open-ended activity plans, such as "I think I'll do some gardening." For all your subconscious knows, you could mean 16 hours. Naturally, it will go into a panic and turn up the pain after 30 minutes to stop you going too far.

Half an hour today, 40 minutes tomorrow, perhaps 45 minutes the following day, is an arrangement your subconscious may find more attractive than an open-ended contract. Once you have made a deal with yourself, never give in early and never get carried away by euphoria and cheat.

By setting reasonable, positive goals you can influence your subconscious and increase the amount of activity you wish to do. Pain sufferers who cope by setting themselves targets know, of course, that they may have good and bad days. Anticipating the troughs when pain can make activity more difficult than usual is an important part of the psychology. It is advisable to prepare yourself by scaling down activity to ride through the trough. If bad pain days mean that you achieve, say, only half your targets, then it is perfectly reasonable to lower them and work up again when you are heading for a peak.

It was all conditioning

One man on a pain management program provided a vivid demonstration of conditioning. Although his original illness had disappeared, he found that a day's work generated a tremendous amount of pain. By the time he got home in the evening and sat in his recliner, the pain was unbearable. On the program, the exercise and physical activity were much greater than at work, yet he felt hardly any pain when he sat down to rest. The culprit turned out to be the recliner, which conditioned his behavior because it had so many pain associations. He threw the chair out and never experienced pain on such an intense level again.

Treatment for Pain Has Evolved

In the 1960s, doctors treated pain on the theory that many conditions could be improved by surgery. If your back hurt, the idea was to "nail" it together again. When that failed to work, the answer was to "nail" it better, harder, bigger. This continued until a realization evolved that the approach was of little permanent help.

The Behavioral Solution

Medical opinion came to the conclusion that there were other reasons that pain patients continued to suffer – pain was multifactorial. Pain came to be viewed as behavior in the way that accent is a kind of behavior. People may speak with a regional accent because those around them spoke the same way when they were children and they felt that it was the best way to behave. Similarly, if a child from, say, Texas immigrated to Canada, he would subtly adopt a Canadian accent as a way of relating to other children. He would not modify his accent on account of his parents – he would feel secure in their love and affection; but because he felt unsure of other children, it would be easier to change and fit in with them.

Ever since Pavlov trained dogs to salivate by associating the sound of a bell with food, doctors have been aware that

---

The School of Bravery

The Japanese developed a behavioral system called "The School of Bravery," in which patients with conditions such as rheumatoid arthritis were made to walk and run. When they were asked how they felt, they replied, "It hurts like hell. But I'm being very brave." Conditioning people to change their behavior is not the whole answer. Motivation has to be made to come from within, by combining positive attitude with exercise, relaxation and an understanding of the psychology of pain.

---

behavior can be changed. The same subconscious conditioned response that made Pavlov's dogs drool can produce pain in people under certain circumstances.

In the 1960s, American pain researchers concluded that if you had acute pain and were off work, receiving sickness benefits and behaving like an invalid, your family took notice of you. You acquired a pain behavior that, in time, might go on to become chronic pain.

Based on the conviction that pain was learned, early programs took the approach of making people unlearn their behavior, which in many ways was not very different from unsophisticated brainwashing. The system, now abandoned in its pure form, has merits when used in other areas. Children in a hospital, for example, may come from homes where they have learned that the only way to get attention is to be naughty. Hospital staff take a behavioral approach by ignoring them when they are naughty and giving them the attention they crave when they are good.

Early pain programs revolved almost entirely around the principle that people would be ignored when they complained of pain. They were told that if they did things positively, they would get attention. If they writhed on the floor in agony, staff would step over them. What's more, they would teach the patient's family to do the same.

The psychology was tough and ultimately in the patient's interest, but constituted only a small part of a complete approach to pain relief. Its shortcoming was that patients were all being tagged with the same behavioral label, when, in fact, their conditions were very diverse.

Pain Management Today – the Cognitive Approach
The modern approach to pain management began when patients on behavioral courses started to talk to psychologists and ask if there weren't other ways of achieving the same ends. One of the first methods of broadening programs was to introduce relaxation, which is a cognitive approach, as opposed to conditioning. Cognition means discovering about ourselves, and it enabled patients to realize that when their backs hurt, they could make themselves more relaxed and therefore feel less pain. "Right attitude" began to play a central role in learning how to manage pain.

The pain management program advocated in this book developed from an awareness that patients were not responding to other treatments, and is based on the belief that patients need to become fit, to relax and to learn more about themselves. As the program evolved, other aspects were accepted, including the importance of certain therapies, some of which were not generally recognized, and the therapeutic value of working in groups.

Patients also needed reassuring that the staff genuinely believed they were in pain – that they were not malingering or complaining for no reason. In turn, patients had to understand that their pain was not simply a physical experience; there were emotional and psychological ramifications that could make it worse. Until they understood that, their condition could not improve. They had to recognize too that they could not rely on drugs, and that if they continued to take large quantities they would feel worse. Removing this psychological crutch was an important step toward learning the right attitude. Combining these lessons and applying them diligently continues to bring about remarkable changes in outlook.

Just how successful this approach can be is illustrated by the case of Betty, who had suffered from back pain since the birth of her daughter in 1974: "During the birth, I was given an epidural that went wrong. Two pieces of catheter broke off in my back, causing severe back pain and a loss of feeling in my leg. Two weeks later, I had an operation in which the surgeon managed to remove one of the pieces. Over the following nine months I had problems with the operation scar, because stitches inserted deep in my back were being rejected and causing an infection. I had to have surgery again to remove all the stitches and clean the wound. These two operations on my spine caused a weakness, in addition to the back pain and loss of feeling in my leg. In the early 1980s I took a job in a warehouse, assembling orders of drugs for pharmacies, but had to leave because my back pain was so severe. Around 1985, an orthopedic surgeon made some attempts to inject cortisone into my spine, but the treatment did not work. He advised my doctor to send me to the pain relief clinic. Various methods of controlling the pain by treating nerve ends and removing scar tissue were tried, but I was finally told that the pain could not be cured.

"At the time I joined the pain management program I was taking lorazepam and naproxen and acetaminophen, when I was in severe pain. My activity was very low. I stayed in bed late in the mornings. I did not go out shopping and did not often visit my friends. At the start of the course I was depressed, fed up, angry, irritable and had lost all my confidence.

"One of the targets I achieved was to go out shopping on my own. I also plan to go out more often socially and visit my family and friends. More than anything, I have changed emotionally and now have a different, positive outlook on life. As a result, I feel happier and not as irritable and angry. My husband and children have noticed a big difference in my attitude. I feel more complete again."

FOUR

The Importance of a Healthy Body – Exercise and Diet

Exercise is one of the most powerful weapons in the fight against pain. Swimming, walking, gentle aerobics and similar activities all release endorphins, which not only help you overcome pain but make exercise fun. They bring about a feeling of well-being that many pain sufferers forget they once possessed. Without exercise, even the fittest of us become depressed.

Here's an example. A doctor was an outstanding athlete as a schoolboy. When he enrolled in medical school he decided that there was no time for both study and sports, and gave up sports. Within three months he became increasingly depressed without understanding the reason, and at one time even contemplated suicide. He was advised that it was because he had given up the exercise that had become an integral part of his life. He worked out a program of jogging to the hospital five mornings a week, not because he was unfit, but to keep himself from becoming depressed. By creating a niche in his life for exercise, he regained his happiness.

Professional athletes, and people who exercise regularly, often become low in spirits if they break a leg and have to stay on the injury list. Star athletes who strain a tendon often feel they will never attain peak form again because they feel depressed at being out of training. They find it hard to believe in themselves when they are laid up. We all have to believe in ourselves, and being unfit through pain takes this away from us.

When you are in pain it is difficult not to be overprotective of yourself. This is reasonable with acute pain – if you break your leg or have angina, you don't try to run upstairs. With chronic pain that is manifestly not the case. In recent years medicine has tended to move away from a negative outlook on pain and recovery and become much more positive. A generation ago, someone recovering from a heart attack would be in the hospital for up to a month. Staff would very gingerly get the person out of bed after three or four days and, frankly, worry about him or her dropping dead.

Twenty years before, the approach was even more cautious. Heart patients were hospitalized for six weeks and confined to bed for half that period, with strict orders not to move. They were warned that their hearts were so bad that when they were finally allowed out of bed, they would be breathless. We realize now, of course, that anyone would be breathless after three weeks in bed, because he or she would be unfit.

Today, heart attack patients are admitted to the hospital and, providing there are no complications, find themselves in a chair the same day. Ten days in the hospital is now not uncommon for heart attack victims.

A similarly progressive view is being taken with orthopedic problems. A decade ago, a soccer player who had to have a knee operation would be in a cast for six weeks, and would then need another six weeks of physiotherapy to break down the adhesions from the cast. A player may now have a knee operation and be playing four weeks later.

When someone has cartilage removed, activity is going to be painful, but doctors take the view that it will certainly do no harm to exercise within a week. Some fractures in children are now not even put in casts. If the child can use his or her arm, and no dislocating force is going to be applied to it, then it is more beneficial to be able to move it around.

Exercise is vital because it helps to overcome pain and fight the depression immobility brings. As the treatment of acute pain has become more aggressive with regard to getting patients quickly back on their feet, the approach to chronic pain needs to move even farther in that direction. The chronic-pain sufferer may have been encouraged by the physician and family not to exercise. Those around the person quickly become oversolicitous with such comments as "Don't do the garden, dear – you might hurt yourself" or "Leave the dishes. I'll do them for you," turning the person into an invalid and making him or her unfit.

A psychologist working at a university was suffering from tension and depression. The problem had begun with sciatica, caused by disk disease in his back. Although it was possible to operate on him, his doctor had decided it might be unwise because he had mild hemophilia and ran the risk of bleeding. When he complained that the pain was terrible, he was advised not to be as active, because it was obviously not good for him.

This was bad news for the psychologist because he and his wife ran a small farm, with five acres of vegetables to till, chickens that needed feeding and a cow that had to be milked twice a day. Afraid of ignoring his doctor's advice, he stopped doing everything, and became very depressed. His wife had twice the amount of work to do and soon there was friction between them, which made him tense and even more depressed.

As a psychologist, he understood his condition – he was under stress because his lifestyle had been changed and he was now afraid to do anything. When he was examined there was no sign of any disk disease he might once have had. It appeared that the surgeon had not wanted to operate because of the psychologist's hemophilia and had advised him to give up physical work as a safety precaution.

The patient was now told there was no evidence that any exercise would harm him in any way and was asked what he really wanted. "All I want," he replied, "is an assurance that I can safely go back and work on my farm." The doctor took a sheet of letterhead stationery and wrote: "You can go back and work on your farm," then handed it to him. "This is exactly what I needed," he said. "Permission for my subconscious to make it happen."

Six months later, he wrote to say that he was happy again, his relationship with his wife was back to normal and he had found renewed energy for his work at the university. All he had ever wanted was permission to exercise, and without this permission his life had fallen apart.

The classic slogan relating to muscle is "Use it or lose it." If you do not exercise there is the strongest likelihood that you will embark on a dreary cycle of depression and pain. Even the healthiest people will have muscle weakness and back pain if they spend most of their time in bed or in a chair.

Get Moving Again in Small Stages

Once you believe that you can exercise safely without harm, the problem is, how do you know how far to go?

First, there is no question of going out and running a personal marathon. Even the fittest athletes suffer from stretching themselves too far. The first step is to set a goal you want to achieve and build up to it by attainable stages. If, for example, you would like to take up swimming again, make your first step going to the pool to float on your back and splash around. Have a little fun in the water before getting out. As much as you desperately want to swim 16 lengths, it is important that you not even try. On your second visit, you could perhaps aim to swim a width, and the next time, two widths. If you find that easy or encouraging, then try a couple of lengths on the following occasion. If that proves too much, revert to widths again until you feel ready for greater things.

The idea is to create your exercise program in tiny units you are sure you can handle. Always aim for the simplest goals to increase your fitness, confidence and well-being. If you do so your progress will always be positive and will move steadily forward.

This gradual approach also applies to psychological adjustment. If an activity has been painful in the past, the thought of repeating it may be daunting. For example, suppose that pain has prevented you from driving your car and the target you have set is to drive to visit some friends. For the first stage, don't even pick up your car keys. Simply walk to the car and sit behind the wheel for a while. It may be a modest goal, but it is the first step toward driving again.

The second time you get in the car, switch on the engine but don't attempt to drive anywhere. On the next occasion, when you are used to the idea of being in charge of a vehicle again, you can drive a short way down the block. Walk home and ask someone else to move the car back for you. To begin with, it is important only to go forward.

Break your target into small steps that are easy to accomplish and log them on a chart so that you can see yourself progressing toward your goal of driving, say, to New York and back. It may take a year, but you are not seeking great leaps of improvement. Far better to stick to a time scale that assures you of success.

Keep Those Muscles and Ligaments Working

With each step, you are making yourself active and taking gentle exercise. If you do not exercise you face two debilitating problems: muscle weakness and shortening of the ligaments. When muscles become weak with underuse, even the slightest form of activity can make you tired. When ligaments shorten and you take up exercise to stretch them, they become inflamed. Both these conditions tend to cause pain, if not at the time, then almost certainly the next day.

Many pain sufferers are not incapable of simple exercise such as mowing the lawn. If they really had to do it, they probably could. What prevents them is retribution fear: the knowledge that they will wake up the next morning feeling miserable because they are in pain.

Yet what this pain indicates is simply aching muscles and ligaments, not a worsening of the original pain. It is something professional athletes feel after every event. The time to notice is when you experience a new pain, or worsening of your pain as you are exercising. If, for example, you take a walk and feel a new pain shooting down your leg, then you are probably right to stop and check with your family physician. You may have intermittent claudication (cramping pain caused by poor circulation), vascular problems or even something wrong with a disk. The point is that this is acute pain that is occurring at the time and preventing you from doing a particular activity. Pain felt the next day simply means that you are unfit; it is harmless and can be overcome.

You may accept this and put the pain in perspective, but the thought remains: is it worth going through it? The answer depends upon how much you wish to improve the quality of your life.

Endorphins Lessen Pain and Improve Attitude

Exercise not only enables you to become fitter and to release

Housework can wait

When pain sufferers complain that they get pain when they go out and enjoy themselves, we often discover that it is equally painful to stay at home and do the housework. If that is the case, and you feel you can tackle only one activity, then go out and enjoy yourself and worry about the housework later. There is little point in doing only housework and not enjoying it, because you are not going to improve. Now and again, it is more important to go out and have fun to improve the quality of your life and your sense of achievement and well-being.

This is not an easy decision to make. Some people frankly prefer to stay at home and do the housework, because they consider it more important. What they are choosing to do is to have their pain and be miserable, rather than have it and, for a few hours, be happy. If pain dominates your life, consider changing your routine and adopting a new approach. If you go out socially, you can still attempt the housework next day. The pain will be the same, but as you work you will feel better within yourself. You will have refused to allow pain to gain the upper hand and will have taken a positive step toward overcoming it.

endorphins, it also improves your self-image. Suddenly, from not being able to drive the car, or swim or dance, you are doing the things you have missed. Even participating in them a little is better than not achieving anything at all.

Those who lack the courage to try are held back by fear and worry. They allow pain to win its battle against them and will continue to feel inadequate, angry and depressed. Activity releases endorphins that not only reduce pain, but make you feel good and give you the confidence to do more.

Having the right attitude actually helps produce endorphins too. Whether your motive is pride, determination or a cussed refusal to be a victim of pain for the rest of your life, you are taking positive steps to gain control of your pain.

Marathon runners face the same problem constantly when, toward the end of a race, they encounter "the wall" – the point at which they are in so much pain that they are desperate to drop out and give up. They know, from experience, that they can either quit or produce endorphins to take them through the barrier and enable them to finish. At that moment, their decision hinges on attitude.

Despite training hard and being exceptionally fit, all marathon runners reach this crisis in a race. What pushes them on is commitment. A football player took part in a marathon and was in such pain that he was on the point of signaling for the ambulance. Ahead of him he saw a man in his sixties, still going on and clearly determined to finish. The player thought, "If he can do it at his age, so can I," and summoned the reserves he needed to cross the finish line.

Once you reach that point, it is as though your subconscious, which has been urging you to play safe and give up, suddenly realizes that you mean business and decides to offer all the help it can. In daily life, your subconscious will always try to persuade you to capitulate to pain because it knows you are afraid of harming yourself. Once you stamp your authority upon it and prove your determination, it will produce the endorphins to carry you through. Afterward, you will feel better – for the same reason that marathon runners are elated when they finish a race. Endorphins not only help you to break through the wall of pain, but make you feel good in the process.

Commitment can take you far

The 400 meters is acknowledged to be one of the most demanding races in athletics. For the first 300 meters, their training carries runners through. At 310 meters they have a burning in their chest not unlike a major heart attack. At this stage, they know that they still have some distance to go. The question they have to ask themselves is whether they can put up with the pain for another 10 seconds. Their subconscious tells them that if they stop, it will go away. Experience tells them that if they listen, their next race will be even more difficult. As soon as they decide to complete the final 90 meters, the pain becomes less important.

Exercising with Others Helps

Like athletes, pain sufferers have to believe in themselves. Working alone is not easy, which is precisely why athletes have coaches to motivate them and give them the incentive to break through the pain. Exercising with others is not only more fun, but more effective.

You don't have to join a keep-fit group for disabled people if you are in pain. Any kind of swimming, walking or exercise group will do, as long as you explain your condition and make it clear to the instructor that you will only be able to work at a low initial rate. The danger of some go-for-the-burn exercise groups is that they encourage participants to work flat out. If you try to compete, there is a real danger of hurting yourself, which is not the right approach when you are in chronic pain.

Build up gradually, and never exercise until you hurt if you suffer chronic pain, or else you will almost certainly damage muscles. When you exercise with others, select your group carefully so that you can obtain maximum benefit. Tai chi and yoga are excellent in this respect. Many community centers now provide exercise for the elderly, passive exercise to music or movement in water (aquarobics).

In groups of this kind you will not feel pressure to keep up, or worry that you are being left behind. It is always important to avoid placing yourself in a negative situation. Other members, who are healthy and not suffering pain, must appreciate that you may be a little slower. Set out your own ground rules before you take part. Explain that you will be swimming only half a length, and after two weeks you hope to be swimming a length. There is no way you will be able to swim 40 lengths with the rest of them.

When they see that you have your own program and targets, people in the group with the right attitude will give all the support they can. The value of joining is that people who care pick you up when you are down. After coping with pain on your own, it is a joy to answer the phone and hear someone say, "We missed you last week. Couldn't you make it?"

All kinds of people, from dieters to alcoholics, know that they receive more support and make more personal progress with understanding people around them. Few people who read this book will be able to overcome pain alone, without any kind of outside assistance. The social aspect of conquering pain is extremely important. If, for example, you are unable to join a relaxation group, then perhaps going to a place of worship and relaxing there would be of some benefit.

Making the effort to get up and go out, to become more active socially, works in harmony with exercise and relaxation. One of the most common problems in the elderly, for instance, is loneliness. Elderly women with back pain who join a pain management program tend to require little treatment. By the end of the third or fourth week, many are laughing as they exercise because there is finally some point in doing it. At home, there seemed to be little incentive.

How You Do It Counts – Not What You Do

Another point to consider about working on muscles and ligaments is that the type of exercise you choose doesn't matter as long as it has value for you. If you are frightened of water, then there is little value in swimming. Some people enjoy ten-pin bowling, and while it may not score high on everyone's list, if it is fun for the sufferers and keeps them active, then it will produce positive results in their fight against pain. Whatever form of exercise you choose, the release of endorphins will be a tangible morale booster.

Gentle exercise will cut down the pain you are suffering. It is not enough for muscles and ligaments that you do the housework or walk around the mall. Exercise programs strengthen muscles that are normally underused, and help to stabilize the spine.

People with arthritis or rheumatism can exercise too

Just as many myths surround pain, there are quite a few fallacies concerning exercise if you suffer from arthritis or rheumatism.

- Your joints do not wear out with overuse! In fact, it is much better to use them than to sit in a chair all day, because this causes stiffness.
- If you find that exercise is causing you pain in your joints, perhaps you are doing too much. Little and often is better than prolonged exercise periods.
- Housework and gardening are fine, in short spells interrupted by short rests.
- When you do sit, don't sit in one place for too long – from time to time get up and stretch your joints.

When you exercise it is important to remember to follow through the full extent of any movement because, quite often, it is the last part of the action that carries the benefit. If you are asked to straighten your arm or stretch your neck, try to follow the instructions as fully as you are able.

Exercise and Myofascial Pain

Exercise is of enormous benefit to patients suffering from myofascial pain, which is caused by muscles developing tender fibrous nodules called *trigger points*. Pressure on these points can give rise to a characteristic aching pain. The problem may be treated by acupuncture, local anesthetic injections, acupressure and "spray and stretch" therapy, which help you perform the exercises that are the key to sustained relief.

Specific exercises that relieve myofascial pain provide a good general warm-up to a sustained exercise program. Basic rules for avoiding myofascial pain are also sound advice to all pain sufferers:

- *Never* bend and lift, or pull something with your back twisted.
- *Always* lift with your knees bent, holding your back in an erect forward-facing position.

- *Never* get up from a chair, or sit down, while leaning forward in a stooped position with your trunk rotated.

Stretching Exercises for Myofascial Pain

These are easy stretching exercises, working from your neck down to your buttocks. They are not comprehensive, but may help people with myofascial pain choose appropriate exercises, and may help other chronic-pain sufferers loosen up before joining an exercise program.

General neck and back stretching:

Sit with your legs straight out, if you can. Bend your body forward, as if to touch your toes. (You could also place both hands behind your head, which also stretches your back.) If you are very stiff, breathe in deeply and let your tummy push you slightly backward. Then, when you breathe out, let the motion carry your body farther forward a little with each breath.

Neck stretching:

Bend your neck forward to touch your chin to your chest. You can combine this with deep breathing, allowing your chin to drop forward a little with each breath. Move your left ear toward your shoulder, with your face facing forward, then repeat on the opposite side. Touch your chin to your left shoulder and do the same on the opposite side. Then move your occiput – the back of your head – toward your left shoulder and repeat for the opposite side. You will find that these exercises stretch the different muscles of your neck.

Shoulder, chest and back stretching:

Stand in a doorway with your arms outstretched on the doorjambs. Lean slightly forward on your toes and take your weight on your arms, stretching up to your chest (pectoral muscles). If you place your arms upward, you will

stretch the lower muscle fibers; placing your arms downward stretches the upper muscle fibers.

To stretch your shoulder muscles, you can put one arm
across the opposite shoulder, as if to scratch your back. Use
your other arm to push your elbow as far as you can toward
the opposite shoulder. Repeat for the opposite arm. Now
try placing an arm behind you and use the opposite arm to
pull it across your back as far as possible.

To stretch your back muscles, hug yourself tightly and
take a deep breath.

Side stretching:
Stand with your legs slightly apart, look straight ahead and
bend slightly to your left. Try to bring your left hand as far
down your thigh as possible. To add further stretch at the
same time, you can place your right arm over your head,
toward the opposite side. Repeat the stretch toward your
right side.

A Four-Week Exercise Program at Home

Exercising with others is preferable to exercising alone, but if
you are unable to join a group, any exercise is better than
none. The four-week exercise program that follows, which
was devised by physiotherapists, provides a good framework.
The aim is to work all your muscles, building up the number
of repetitions of each movement as the program progresses.

Remember, there is no hurry. You should avoid speed or
sudden jerky movements. Exercise is fun and the objective is
to feel better afterward. The number in brackets after each
movement is a guide to how many times it may be repeated
the first time you exercise.

Standing and Sitting Exercises

Touch toes: If you find you can't reach your toes, extend as far as you comfortably can (*3 times*).

Alternate knee bend: In a standing position, lift your knee as high as you can toward your chest (*5 times*).

Lateral bending: Stand and bend your upper body sideways until it is at right angles to your legs (*5 times*).

Arm circle: Stand and make the biggest circle possible with one arm, then repeat with the other (*5 times*).

Step-ups: Step on and off the first step of your stairs. If you happen to live in a bungalow, try the back-door step or a low bench instead (*5 times*).

Wall slide: Stand with your back against a smooth wall. Slide down into a squatting position, stand up and repeat (*5 times*).

Push-ups against the wall: Stand facing a wall, an arm's length away from it. Place your hands against the wall at chest height. Lean forward and slowly push yourself away until your arms are straight (*5 times*).

Forward stretch: Stand and place one foot on a chair or stool. Lean forward to stretch your leg and back muscles (*5 times*).

Stand/sit: Sit on a chair, stand and sit down again (*5 times*).

Chair push-ups: Sit in a chair and push on the arms to raise your bottom from the seat (*5 times*).

Lying Face Up

Ankles up and down: Raise your leg about a hand's width and move your foot forward and backward (*5 times*).

Ankle circling: Raise your leg about a hand's width and rotate your foot (*5 times*).

Alternate straight raises: Raise your leg as high as you can, keeping it straight. Repeat with the other leg (*3 times*).

Lying Knees Bent, Feet on the Mat
Flatten back: When we lie down we tend to have an arch in our lower back. Move your pelvis until the whole of your back makes contact with the floor (*5 times*).
Alternate hand to knee: Touch your left knee with your right hand and then repeat, right hand to left knee (*5 times*).
Alternate arm stretch: Lie with your arms at your sides and raise each arm in turn, stretching as high as you can (*5 times*).

Lying on Right Side, Then Left Side
Leg Raise: Raise your leg vertically as high as you can manage (*3 times*).

Lying Face Down
Alternate leg raise: Try to lift one leg, then the other (*3 times*).
Push-ups: Place your palms on the floor, on either side of your chest, and push yourself up until your arms are straight. Start by keeping the knees bent (*3 times*).

Muscle Tension and Pain

Being unfit and being tense go hand in hand. Most patients arrive at a pain clinic both out of condition and suffering from obvious muscle tension. This is quite understandable, because pain changes their posture, making their muscles work harder to hold the shape that their pain has dictated. Some people are bent over, others twisted into positions that they believe give them less discomfort. When they try to sit straight it hurts because their ligaments have become shortened. To stay in the position shaped by their pain means using certain groups of muscles much harder than others. The result is that some muscles are taut and in constant tension, while others are weak and underused. Most people are unaware of these muscle spasms.

In addition, they are suffering from the anxiety and stress

Muscle spasms hurt!

An anesthetic called succinyl choline is used in operating rooms for certain surgical procedures. It makes all the muscles go into spasm for a few seconds until they burn up energy, exhaust themselves and then totally relax.

It is not unusual for patients who have this anesthetic, especially those with good muscles, to present themselves at a hospital emergency room 24 or 48 hours later with all the signs of a heart attack. They complain of chest pains and turn very pale, and if the hospital is unaware of their operation, staff quite easily think the patient has had a heart attack. The condition wears off in a few days, but at the time it is very real and severe pain is caused by muscle contraction.

of their new lives as invalids. They worry about their futures, their incomes, relationships with their families, as well as how pain is affecting them physically and mentally. Such problems are enough to make anyone tense, but for chronic-pain sufferers this has become a way of life, and many never even realize that their muscles are not relaxed.

Quite often, they say that pain prevents them from leading normal lives because they feel so tired all the time. On examination, it is often found that they are fatigued because their muscles are constantly working at full stretch to no useful end. Many people think that muscle tension cannot be anything serious. You raise your arm horizontally, tensing the muscles, and it does not particularly hurt. Try to hold your arm in that position for five minutes, however, and it becomes agony.

Relaxation, in the sense of having conscious control over your muscles, is an important part of exercise. Engaging in physical activity and then simply allowing your muscles to slacken and rest is not enough. That has the same effect as sitting in front of the TV after a day's work. You think you are relaxed, but your muscles can be tense while your subconscious drifts from one negative thought to another. What has really happened is that your conscious mind has taken a vacation.

For a healthy diet
- Eat a variety of foods.
- Maintain a healthy weight.
- Eat less fat and watch the types of fat.
- Eat plenty of starchy foods, especially those high in fiber.
- Eat plenty of fruit, vegetables and salads.
- Eat less sugar.
- Drink alcohol only in moderation.

Managing pain is being in control, whether doing exercise or relaxing. If you are doing nothing, you are giving pain an opportunity to regain control. Real relaxation involves your conscious mind telling the rest of your body exactly how it wants it to be. Learning to relax means closing the door on pain, even when you are at rest. This is one example of having an internal locus of control.

Diet

Inactivity caused by chronic pain may lead to obesity and other complications, such as osteoarthritis, which is more likely to develop in people who are overweight. Other weight-related problems include high blood pressure, diabetes, gall bladder disease, breathing problems and varicose veins. Choosing to eat a healthy diet not only helps you to control your weight, but may also prevent a number of other health problems that are common in the Western world, including heart disease and stroke, dental caries (tooth decay), bowel disorders and certain cancers.

It is recommended that a variety of foods be eaten because this reduces the risk of any nutritional deficiencies. While you can live on a few foods and have a very healthy diet, unless you have some knowledge of nutrition it may be by luck rather than by design. Many of the so-called cure-all diets, often advocated in magazines, can lead to nutrition problems.

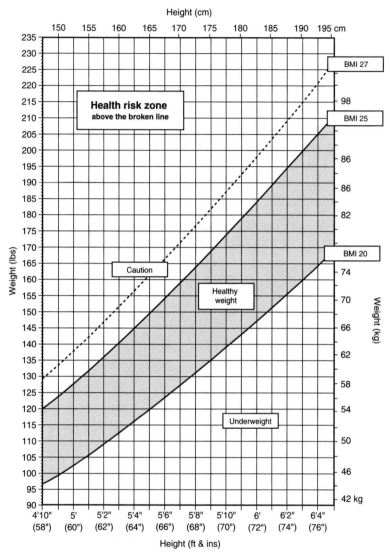

Adapted from Nutrition Services, Ottawa-Carleton Health Department, 1987

Maintain a Healthy Weight

How Do You Know If You Are Overweight?

Most people know whether they are overweight or putting on weight, but it is wise to have an occasional weight check to ensure

If you are overweight, how can you lose weight?

- Reduce your fat and sugar intake.
- Avoid snacking between meals.
- Avoid or reduce alcohol intake.
- Eat plenty of high-fiber foods, including fruit and vegetables.

that your weight is not creeping up. It is always easier to lose a little weight than to mount a long-term campaign to reduce.

If you embark on a diet, it is important to take into account individual food preferences, family habits and social customs. In the West we are spoiled by all the choice we have when shopping for our meals, a point for which we should be grateful. No food is truly "junk," though if eaten in excess some foods are unhealthy. If you are interested in the nutritional content of the food you buy, get into the habit of reading labels. Many of the big food chains produce helpful pamphlets on nutritional topics, including food labeling.

If You Are Underweight, Does It Matter?

If the body mass index (BMI) chart indicates that you are underweight, discuss this with your doctor. Maybe you have no appetite, or you may be eating foods that give you insufficient energy. If there is a problem, your doctor may refer you to a dietitian for advice.

Eat Less Fat and Watch the Types of Fat

Because fat is high in calories, eating too much of it will lead to obesity. A high-fat diet may also sometimes be associated with certain types of cancers. Too much saturated fat, found in meat and dairy foods, is linked to a higher risk of heart and artery disease because it may increase the cholesterol (a type of fat) in the blood. Using small amounts of polyunsaturated fats like fish oils, sunflower oil, corn oil, etc., and monoun-

To reduce fat intake

- Use less butter or margarine. Spread it thinly, or use low-fat spread. Polyunsaturated margarines have the same calories as butter and should be used sparingly if you are dieting.
- Change to nonfat or low-fat milk.
- Try to eat less full-fat cheese and use low-fat cheese or cottage cheese instead. Avoid eating cheese between meals.
- Use low-fat yogurt, sour cream and salad dressings.
- Cut down on high-fat snacks – potato chips, chocolate, cakes, biscuits, pastries.
- Avoid fried foods – grill, microwave, boil, poach, bake or steam instead.
- Eat more fish. All fish is good for you, especially the oily varieties, such as salmon, mackerel and herring.
- Use more chicken or turkey, but avoid the skin because most of the fat is there.
- Buy lean cuts of meat and trim off any visible fat. Eat fewer burgers and sausages, or try to buy "lower-fat" varieties. Eat smaller portions of meat and add more vegetables, including beans, peas or barley, to stews.
- Skim the fat off stews and soups by removing it with paper towels, or chill them and remove the fat when cold.
- Limit eggs to five a week (fewer if you have a cholesterol problem).
- Avoid french fries and roast potatoes – eat boiled or baked potatoes instead, preferably in their skins.
- Use lemon juice or vinegar on salads instead of salad dressing and mayonnaise.
- Avoid high-fat ice cream products. Some low-fat and even fat-free iced desserts are available; read the labels.

saturated fats like olive oil and rapeseed (canola) oil, may help reduce blood cholesterol levels.

If you are not overweight, you are still advised to limit your fat intake. For baking, you could use either margarines high in polyunsaturates or olive oil spreads. For sauces and salad dressings, use an oil high in polyunsaturates or monounsaturates. Always use a suitable oil for frying and do not reuse it more than twice. It is advisable to cut down on french fries; when you do have them, slice them thickly. If you buy frozen french fries, choose those cooked in sunflower or similar oil. Cut down on the amount of potato chips you eat and buy only those cooked in sunflower-type oils.

Eat Plenty of Starchy Foods

These provide the energy for your diet. Unless you are over-weight and advised to limit (not avoid) these foods, they should be taken in good amounts. Starchy foods high in fiber will help to regulate your bowels and some may help reduce your blood cholesterol. If you are prone to constipation – a frequent problem if you take painkillers containing codeine or similar preparations – a high-fiber diet may be particularly beneficial, as well as a high fluid intake.

Which starchy foods should you choose?

- Eat plenty of bread, especially whole-wheat or fiber-enriched.
- Eat more boiled or baked potatoes, preferably in their skins.
- Include breakfast cereals, especially whole-grain varieties such as oatmeal, shredded wheat, muesli, bran flakes and oat cereals.
- Eat more rice, especially brown rice.
- Try more pasta, especially the whole-wheat varieties.
- If you are baking, buy whole-wheat flour. If you find it difficult to use, try using half white and half whole wheat.
- Move over to more peas, beans and lentils. Canned beans and other legumes are easy to use because they do not require soaking and prolonged cooking.

More Fruit, Vegetables and Salads

Apart from providing fiber in your diet, these foods help to give you essential vitamins and minerals, and are thought to cut the risk of heart disease and reduce blood cholesterol levels.

Less Sugar

As well as helping to increase your weight, a high-sugar diet is associated with dental decay and gum disease. All forms of sugar – sucrose, dextrose, glucose, fructose, as well as honey, syrup, raw sugar, brown sugar, cane sugar and caramel – should be avoided where possible.

- Buy fruit canned in its own juice, instead of in syrup.
- Avoid frosted or honey-coated breakfast cereals.
- Cut down on candies, chocolates, cakes and cookies.
- Choose sugar-reduced jams.

Alcohol in Moderation

A high alcohol intake may lead to serious health problems. Since some pain is relieved by alcohol, great care must be taken not to overindulge.

It is suggested, unless you have been advised by your doctor to take less, that low-risk drinking levels are: *men:* no more than two standard drinks per day, with at least one day a week when no alcohol is consumed; *women:* less than men; a small woman should limit herself to one drink per day.

A standard drink is

- 12 ounces (341 mL) normal-strength beer or cider;
- 1.5 ounces (45 mL) of spirits;
- 5 ounces (145 mL) of wine.

Whatever your intake within these limits, always have alcohol with food; and carefully read the labels of off-the-shelf or prescribed drugs – they may advise against taking alcohol.

To Sum Up

Adequate exercise and a proper diet are essential in controlling pain. Remember:

- Exercise daily.
- Aim for realistic goals.
- Follow a realistic exercise program.
- You are what you eat.

Mastering Relaxation

Years of pain research and the experience of hundreds of doctors working in pain management indicate that it is almost impossible to have chronic pain without having muscle spasm. No matter how relaxed you may feel, you almost certainly have tightness of the muscles linked to the area of pain.

Even if you believe that you do not need to learn how to relax, the physiological facts state otherwise. Pain, as we have seen, causes sufferers to lose their locus of control, so that pain takes them over and dictates their lives. Relaxation is the trigger to regaining lost control. It is easy to learn, but requires months of patience and a determination to put time aside each day to make it work.

The Purpose of Muscle Spasms

Pain and muscle spasms go hand in hand. The reaction of a muscle to injury or discomfort is faster than the process of thought. It does not come from the conscious mind, or even the subconscious, but works with such instantaneous speed that pain can occur within a fraction of a second of an injury.

If you put your hand on a hot stove element, for example, you do not go through a reasoning process. It is not a case of a nerve message reaching your brain and telling you that you are in pain and that it would be wise to remove your hand. What happens is that you snatch away your hand before you are even conscious that anything has happened. The pain is not felt until after the muscles have contracted. This is an important mechanism to understand. The muscles contract as a protective reaction even before you know you are in pain. They jerk to pull you away from the source of the pain as fast as possible.

We all know that this is what happens in acute situations, such as burning yourself or pricking your finger. In the case of internal pain, the muscles go into spasm around the area to make that particular part of your body rest. If you break your leg, muscles go into spasm to create a natural splint. Similarly with appendicitis, the muscles of the abdomen go as rigid as a board, which is one of the signs medical students are taught to look for when diagnosing it.

You have no control over this. Muscle spasm is a reflex reaction. Yet it is not always a helpful one. If you dislocate your shoulder an intense muscle spasm locks around it to keep it immobile. Patients have to be sedated to have their shoulders manipulated back into place. On many occasions, as soon as the muscle relaxant has taken effect and their muscles are relaxed, the shoulder slips back into position almost of its own accord.

Muscle Spasms Serve No Useful Purpose in Chronic Pain
At times muscle spasm can be useful, but occasionally it can have no practical use whatever. In almost every case of chronic pain, the muscle spasm accompanying it is useless. Sufferers don't want to be forced to rest. They need to be active to overcome their pain, but muscle tension prevents this, giving rise to many problems. The pain and discomfort of needlessly tense

muscles can induce anxiety and depression and make you tense as a person.

What complicates the matter for many chronic-pain sufferers is that if they have been tense for 10 years, they are no longer aware of it. Many people adamantly claim that they have no need to learn relaxation, when their physiological signs clearly say otherwise.

In the cycle of pain, muscle tension leads to more pain, fear of future pain, bad posture, lack of sleep, more muscle tension – and so it goes on. Unless chronic-pain patients unlock their muscle tension, there is every possibility of their general health becoming worse. Sitting in front of the TV or knitting does nothing to relieve reflex muscle tension. The only way to make positive progress is to learn one of the various methods of conscious relaxation, and to tell your body and your subconscious exactly what you want them to do.

Chronic pain has a life of its own, even when the original illness or damage has disappeared. Chronic muscle spasms can result from an acute injury, such as tearing a muscle, injuring a nerve root or breaking a bone. Even when the original injury has healed, or the nerve has recovered, or the bone has mended, the spasm can remain. The pain continues to be generated along the same nerve pathways, but from a different cause.

Sometimes people hurt their backs at work, or suffer a whiplash injury in a car, and when their doctor examines them nothing wrong is found, but the pain still persists. The doctor may diagnose a muscle spasm but feels, in all fairness, that the acute injury is no longer present. There may no longer be anything physically wrong with the person, but the pain continues to be disabling and real.

People with arthritis may find that their arthritis disappears, but the pain is maintained by muscle spasm. Occasionally, there may not even have been any physical disease at all – the whole

HOW CHRONIC PAIN DEVELOPS

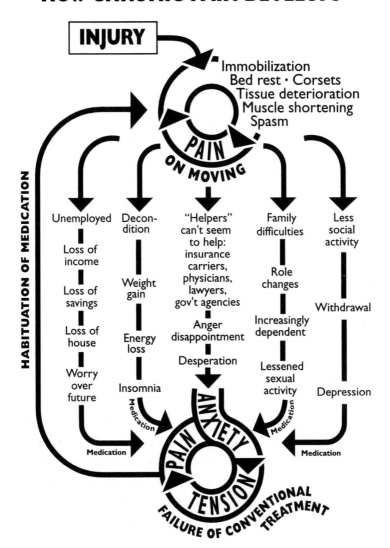

problem may have been caused by muscle spasm in the first place.

Tension affects the muscles and organs of the body and can give rise to such alarming symptoms as headaches, pains elsewhere, sweating, insomnia, indigestion and heart palpitations, which in turn can increase alarm and anxiety. A tense muscle is a painful one. It limits and restricts your movement, makes you feel tired, irritable and unable to concentrate or think clearly.

Relieve Muscle Tension with Relaxation

Relaxation is the opposite of tension – a method of exercise that can help you overcome the physical and emotional suffering of muscle tension. It is a skill and, as with all skills, practice makes perfect. Once you have learned the technique, you can relax anytime, anywhere, and ease the pressure on your body and mind.

The difficult aspect is that relaxation is not like riding a bicycle. Once you have learned it, it does not come automatically. It is important to be aware of some of the problems and remember them at times when you feel that your progress is slow.

On occasion, there have been patients who have mastered the art of relaxation and no longer need to put it into practice; the knowledge that they can control their own muscles is sufficient to keep their pain at a reduced level. For them, such knowledge has provided a feeling of security, like carrying a spare tire in your car. If you know you have one, the prospect of a flat tire poses no worry. If you have no means of dealing

---

The benefits of relaxation

Relaxation is not easy, but some people pick it up more effortlessly than others. The advice from anyone who practices relaxation regularly is to stick with it – the benefits can literally change your life.
Relaxation

- relieves the spasm of a muscle;
- releases endorphins to relieve pain;
- helps you regain your locus of control. If you can learn to relax and reduce your pain, even to a small degree, you are in control again. Once you can control your pain it assumes a totally different perspective. It no longer controls you and confidence takes over from fear and anxiety.

with it, then the thought preoccupies you and assumes an importance that it does not deserve.

What's the Best Method of Relaxation?

All have advantages and disadvantages and the devotees of one method may criticize another. The technique with the greatest chance of success is the one that feels most comfortable to you. There are many: meditation, hypnosis, yoga, tai chi, the tense-and-relax method, visualization.

Preference may depend on many things. Some cultures already have disciplines that tend to draw them to relaxation naturally. Yoga is an accepted part of the Hindu lifestyle; millions of Chinese practice tai chi in their local parks each morning; Muslims pray five times every day. All these combine physical movement and focusing the mind.

In the West, traditional safety mechanisms have been eroded. Church attendance has declined, the friendly corner druggist who would listen to your troubles and "mix a good bottle" has been replaced by self-service drugstores. Even the opportunity to share problems in a doorstep chat with a neighbor has become less common. By turning to drugs and doctors instead, we have lost something of the art of unloading tension. Relaxation does not come easily, so it is important to find a way of achieving it that feels comfortable to you.

"The technique most useful for someone learning to relax is progressive muscular relaxation," says neuropsychologist Dr. Eric Ghadiali. "The principle is that you focus progressively on each muscle group of the body, first tensing as hard as you can and noticing what it actually feels like when it is tensed, then letting go and experiencing how it feels for that particular muscle group to be relaxed.

"Sometimes, when people have particular pain conditions,

Create a daily relaxation routine

- Put aside half an hour each day to devote to relaxation.
- Tell your family and friends what you are doing so they do not interrupt you. Once they know how serious you are, they will provide valuable encouragement and support.
- Choose the same bed, mat or chair each day for your relaxation. A routine helps to settle your mind and put you in a more relaxed state for the exercise.

---

tensing the muscle may bring on the pain. If that is the case, the advice is simply not to tense that particular muscle.

"The advantage of the technique is that it is easy. It is also recognized as one of the quickest ways of teaching people how to relax by increasing your awareness of when you become tense and how you are when relaxed.

"The other main method is autogenic training, when you direct your attention to different muscles groups and concentrate on relaxing thoughts. Instead of thinking how much pain you have, how bad it feels and how awful things are, you focus on a particular muscle instead. Your thoughts are that it is feeling very heavy, very comfortable, very loose, very limp. By doing this progressively – moving from one muscle group to the next – you will be able to relax yourself.

"One of the difficulties people encounter is that they cannot concentrate. The pain becomes too intrusive and takes their attention away. They may even be worried about making dinner, or what time their partner is arriving home from work. The message here is to stick with it. Keep trying to relax, even though you may not feel better in the early stages. Remember that it is a skill and you will gradually improve."

Proper Breathing Is a Must
Coping with pain requires a different lifestyle and new routines, jettisoning old, unhelpful habits and acquiring new ones

that encourage positive progress. Learning how to breathe properly so you can relax is one new habit.

When you are sitting or lying comfortably it is essential to breathe in a calm way. Be careful not to breathe too deeply – taking very deep breaths can sometimes make you feel a little more tense.

The preferred method is to sit or lie with a straight spine. After a full exhalation, inhale through your nose while counting slowly to four. As you inhale, first fill the lower section of your lungs. Your diaphragm will push your abdomen outward to make room for the air.

Then fill the middle part of your lungs as your lower ribs and chest move forward to accommodate more air. Next fill the upper part of your lungs. As you raise your chest and shoulders slightly, draw in your abdomen a little to support your lungs. With practice, these three steps can be performed in one smooth, continuous operation.

Hold your breath for a slow count of three. Exhale through your mouth, making a relaxing, whooshing sound, like wind, as you blow out to a slow count of four. As you exhale, follow the same pattern as the inhalation. Pull your abdomen in, then exhale from your middle chest. Finally, exhale from your upper chest as you allow your shoulders to sink and relax and your abdomen to puff out again slightly.

Not everyone is a natural "belly breather" and the rhythm may be difficult for you to get into. It may help while learning to place one hand lightly on your chest and the other on your abdomen to feel them rise and fall as you inhale and exhale. As the sequence becomes automatic, you can return your hands to a more comfortable position. Scan your body for areas of tension, and return to the sound and flow of your breathing as you become more and more relaxed.

Continue this for five minutes. If you become lightheaded

at any time, alternate six regular breaths with six deep breaths. Once you have learned the breathing exercise, you can practice it whenever you feel yourself becoming tense.

Always try to begin your relaxation session with breathing exercises to put yourself in a calm frame of mind. The important thing is to breathe gently and regularly, feeling your body relax in the process.

Progressive Muscle Relaxation

These simple exercises, which take about 20 minutes, will help you cope with your pain more effectively. They are based on widely used and well-established techniques that are known to help people relax. As we've said, learning how to relax is like learning any new skill – the more you practice, the better you become. Initially, it is recommended that you try these exercises at least every day, more often if you can manage it. Don't worry if you find it difficult at first or don't seem to be succeeding. The trick is not to try too hard.

The exercises you are about to go through will help you to relax all the muscles in your body. They involve repetition, but the rhythm created is part of the beneficial process. During the session you will be progressively tensing, then relaxing, all your muscles. While you are doing this, concentrate on the difference between tension and relaxation.

It is obviously impossible to do these exercises by constantly consulting the book. Either get someone to read you the instructions – it is good for a friend or family member to take part – or, if no one is available, read them into a tape recorder and play them back.

The Basic Method

First, close your eyes. Concentrate on the sound of your breathing. Breathe slowly and regularly, not too deeply. Begin to notice how every time you breathe out you gradually begin to feel more relaxed and more comfortable.

1. Start the muscle relaxation by concentrating on the muscles in your hands, wrists and lower arms. You can tense these by squeezing your hands into fists. Now clench your fists and feel the tension in the muscles. Clench them even tighter and feel the tension – and relax. Let go of the tension. Enjoy the feeling of letting go. Notice the difference between tension and relaxation, how the muscles in your hands and your lower arms feel very loose, very limp, very relaxed.

2. And now the muscles at the front of your upper arms. You can tense these by bending your arms at the elbows and trying to touch your wrists to your shoulders. Bend your arms at the elbows and notice the tension at the front of your upper arms. Make the muscles tight – feel the tension. Tighter – and relax. Let your arms fall to your sides and go loose. Let all the tension go and notice the difference between tension and relaxation – how all the muscles in your arms now feel very loose, limp and relaxed.

3. Now the muscles at the back of your upper arms. You can tense these by straightening out your arms in front of you and making them as stiff as you can. Straighten your arms. Feel the muscles become tense, tenser; feel the tension, hold it – and relax. Let your arms fall to your sides. Concentrate on the difference between tension and relaxation as all the muscles in your arms relax. Notice how your arms now feel very heavy and comfortable. All the muscles in your arms are now very loose, limp and deeply relaxed.

4. Turn your attention now to the muscles in your shoulders. You can tense these by shrugging as tightly as you can. Bring your shoulders up into your neck. Feel the tension. Tense your shoulder muscles as much as you can. Tight,

tighter – feel the tension – and relax. Allow your shoulders to droop and relax. Feel the difference between tension and relaxation as all the muscles in your shoulders relax. Notice how the tension eases as you let the muscles unwind. Notice how all the muscles in your shoulders now feel very loose, very limp and very deeply relaxed.

5. Now for the muscles in your neck. It is easy to tense these muscles by pressing your head back against the chair or bed you are resting on. Press your head backward and feel the muscles becoming very tense and very tight. Experience the tension – and relax. Let your head return to a comfortable position. Concentrate on the difference between tension and relaxation as you let go, and feel all the muscles in your neck become loose, limp and deeply relaxed. Notice how, as all your muscles become more relaxed, you feel more comfortable.

6. Concentrate now on the muscles in your face, starting with the muscles in your forehead. You can tense these by lifting your eyebrows as though in an expression of surprise. Lift your eyebrows as high as you can. Hold it. Feel the tension. Concentrate on the tension in the muscles in your forehead – and relax. Think about the difference between tension and relaxation in your forehead muscles. Let your eyebrows relax. Notice the skin across your forehead and scalp as it becomes very smooth, very loose, very limp and deeply relaxed. There is no tension. You feel much more comfortable as you become more and more deeply relaxed.

7. Next come the muscles around your eyes and face. These can be tensed by squeezing your eyes shut and frowning as hard as you can. Feel the pressure in your eyelids and the tension around your eyes and forehead. Focus on the tension. Make the muscles tight – tighter – and relax. Feel the difference as your muscles unwind and the tension

flows away, leaving all the muscles in your eyes and fore-head loose and deeply relaxed.

8. Now for the muscles in your mouth and jaw. Clamp your teeth together and clench your jaw. Feel the tension build in your mouth and jaw. Hold it, feel the pressure and relax. Let your teeth part slightly and you will notice the difference between tension and relaxation as the muscles in your mouth and jaw go loose and limp. As you become more and more deeply relaxed, so you become more comfortable. Notice now how all the muscles in your lips, face and forehead feel very smooth, heavy and comfortable. Your arms feel very heavy, limp and relaxed. You are breathing slowly and regularly. Every time you breathe out, you feel a greater sense of well-being and comfort.

9. And now the muscles in your chest. These can be tensed by breathing in as deeply as you can. Fill your lungs, breathe very deeply and hold it. Feel the tension in your chest increase and the muscles in your chest become tense. Hold it until it begins to feel uncomfortable – and relax. Feel all the muscles in your chest relax as you breathe out. Continue breathing normally. Not too deeply, but regularly and evenly. Notice the feeling in your chest and the difference between tension and relaxation. The muscles in your chest now feel very comfortable and relaxed.

10. Now focus on the muscles in your stomach. You can tense these by pulling your stomach in tightly, as if preparing to receive a blow. Make your stomach as tight and tense as you can. Feel the tension tightening. Hold it – and relax. Let go of all the tension in your stomach muscles. Notice how they feel very loose, comfortable and deeply relaxed.

11. Now the muscles in your legs. You can tense these by stretching your legs out in front of you, making them stiff and straight and pointing your toes away from your head.

Feel the tension throughout your legs. Tighten all the muscles – tighter – and relax. Let your legs and feet return to a comfortable position. Notice the difference between tension and relaxation in all the muscles of your legs and feet and the way they now feel very heavy, very loose and deeply relaxed.

All the muscles in your body now feel very limp and comfortable. Your whole body feels heavier as you feel yourself sinking deeper into the chair or bed that you are lying on. As you sink deeper, you become more relaxed and comfortable. Your legs are heavy and deeply relaxed. Your hands and arms are very loose. All the muscles in your chest and stomach are very limp and relaxed. The muscles in your forehead, your face, your lips and mouth are very loose and comfortable.

Spend the next few moments focusing on how pleasant and comfortable you feel. You may find it helpful to imagine a relaxing scene or an idyllic scene from your past, perhaps sitting in a warm, sunny garden or lying on a beach listening to the sound of the waves.

Finish the exercise by counting backward from four to one. As you open your eyes you will feel more refreshed and alert, while remaining comfortable and relaxed. As you keep up with the exercises, you will find yourself generally more interested in what you are doing, calmer, more settled, more confident about doing what you want to do and much more in control of your pain.

As you become more accomplished at relaxation, you can use the time at the end of an exercise to plan how to cope with things that might arise during the day. Practice relaxation while going about your daily activities, so that no muscle tension creeps in to give you pain afterward.

An Alternative Method
Breathing

Try to achieve a slow and steady breathing pattern using your diaphragm. The top part of your chest should stay fairly still, and your stomach should slowly rise as you breathe in and fall as you breathe out.

Face

1. Raise your eyebrows, hold, lower them.
2. Push your eyebrows toward your nose, hold, release them.
3. Clench your lips and teeth, hold, then release.
4. Check that your tongue is not pressed hard against the roof of your mouth.

Neck

1. Press your head down into the pillow, hold and release. Let your head rest gently on the pillow.
2. Raise your head slightly off the pillow, hold and release.

Shoulders

Push your shoulders up toward your ears, hold and release. Notice how they fall into a lower position.

Arms

1. Lift your arms half an inch (about a centimeter) off the floor. Make your elbows straight. Hold and release.
2. Leaving your arms supported on the mat, spread your fingers out away from you. Hold and release.

Stomach

Pull your stomach in toward you, hold and release. Notice how difficult breathing is when your stomach is tense.

Buttocks

Clench your buttocks. Feel them lift slightly off the floor; hold and then release.

Legs
1. Push your ankles and toes down, away from your body. Make your knees straight. Hold and release.
2. Let your hips and knees roll out slightly and your feet flop to the side (like 10 minutes to 2 on the hands of a clock).
3. Pull your ankles and toes in toward you, hold and release.

Your body may feel quite heavy now and you should feel calm and at ease. Lie there, savoring the sensation, and notice the difference between how tense you were previously and the way you feel at present. This quick relaxation technique should be used to supplement the longer method previously described, not instead of it. It could be done, for instance, just before or just after doing your physical exercise routine.

Regaining Emotional Control through Relaxation

Relaxation is about regaining control through a new awareness of your body, but not all tension is caused by muscle spasm. There can be many other sources of tension in life that arise as secondary consequences of pain.

"Pain makes people irritable," says Dr. Ghadiali. "It makes them bad-tempered, stops them mixing with their family and friends, makes them touchy. When people are like that, these bad feelings can sometimes be infectious and make the whole family feel uptight – and that can be an additional source of stress. If you can avoid these effects or deal with them in a different way, you can reduce your tension. If you don't recognize them or deal with them, they will still be there, building additional tension.

"These exercises might take 20 minutes, so when you devote half an hour a day to relaxation, try to spend the rest of the time thinking ahead to how you respond to stressful situations with that buildup of tension. Some people clench their teeth when they are in an argument, for example. In a traffic jam they clench their hands or hunch their shoulders when driving. Try to become more aware of how tense you are in everyday situations. Then, instead of responding in the usual way, you can respond by breathing properly and applying your relaxation techniques.

"The secret is increased awareness. In a way, you are conditioning yourself. When you are tense in certain situations, the idea is to decondition yourself and break the association between stressful situations and feeling tense, and so replace the tension with a relaxed reaction."

Many chronic-pain patients find relaxation a difficult knack to learn because they do not know what they are looking for. Some have no idea what a relaxed muscle feels like and nothing to compare it with. When they do begin to acquire relaxation skills, it is usually sitting in a comfortable chair or lying on a mat.

If you have, say, a whiplash injury and are frightened of getting behind the wheel of your car again, then putting relaxation into practice is a different proposition from listening to a soothing tape in an armchair. You must be prepared to broaden your relaxation methods and apply different techniques to your own particular problem. You may have to sit at home and visualize situations: driving in heavy traffic, turning from left to right, shifting the gears and learning to relax your muscles in all these situations before embarking on them. Eventually, you need to be able to relax even in the most stressful situations, such as driving in traffic jams when late or being told unpleasant news.

If you really want to be active again, these are the levels you should aim for. They may take six months or even two years to achieve, but if you are prepared to put in the time and effort, the results are worth it.

Determination Pays Off

One patient ran a family hotel. She had had a slipped disk, which had been successfully treated, but she continued to suffer pain from muscle spasm. Because of her disability, she had to employ three additional staff to continue her work in the hotel.

She worked hard at following the pain management program and had the right positive attitude, but failed to make much progress. Despite taking in all the ideas, she returned to the clinic at a later date to complain that she was still in pain. Her back muscles were still locked in spasm and we knew only relaxation could be of any benefit.

She had learned the technique in the program, but had been able to make little progress. We reviewed the method and she went back to the hotel and continued to practice relaxation every day. After a while, she reported some improvement; she was able to walk around more, but still could not undertake difficult jobs, such as making the beds.

Four and a half years later, after persisting every day, she mastered the knack of relaxing her muscles at will and reliev-

---

Break the vicious tension–pain cycle

Chronic pain causes all kinds of psychological distress, leading to a vicious cycle of tension and more pain. Relaxation techniques are a helpful way of breaking the cycle and reducing tension pain.

- Relax daily – 30 minutes of the method of your choice.
- Visualize different situations at the end of the exercise and how you might cope.
- Remember your internal locus of control – "I am in control here."
- Think positively about the future – "I *will* be able to do this."

ing the pain. "Most of my pain has gone away," she wrote triumphantly. "I still get pain when I try to do things, but I can handle it. My greatest joy has been learning to relax my back muscles. It has enabled me to work again."

Through practice she achieved a new awareness of herself that enabled her to cope with her pain. No matter how long it may take you to acquire the skill, whether it be weeks or years, the freedom it rewards you with repays the effort.

There are occasions when it may take a great effort to put the time aside for relaxation, you may find concentration difficult, pain demands your attention or depletes your energy. No matter how low you feel, always try to make the effort. The close link between body and mind means that the very motions of preparing yourself for relaxation and going through the exercise will affect your outlook and improve your sense of well-being. The response to pain and its associated problems of tension and depression is to do something. The framework and routine of relaxation and exercise provide a reliable, positive method of making progress toward conquering your pain. Determination to reclaim your life and never again allow pain to conquer you is the strongest weapon in your armory.

SIX

Thinking, Feeling, Doing

Pain, as we have seen, is about receiving messages. Most kinds of pain contain a physical element, a signal sent out from within the body warning that something is wrong. The brain acts as a radio receiver with an emergency frequency constantly open, listening for distress messages.

We all tune in to our pain frequency differently. Some of us have the volume turned down low because we are not expecting anything; others have it high because we are always anticipating trouble. It's like the yachtsman who takes his boat out for the weekend. Once at sea, he turns on his shortwave radio and leaves it tuned to the coast-guard channel. If the weather is calm, he will probably have the volume low because the chance of any warnings being transmitted is slight. If a storm is expected, he will have his receiver on full volume, alert for emergency and distress messages.

Pain has two major aspects – the physical and psychological. The psychological, or mental, side does not cause pain, but acts as a volume control, turning the intensity up or down. Like the yachtsman, when the volume is high you receive a

---

Diversionary tactics

An office building had only four elevators. They were hopelessly inadequate to carry the hundreds of office workers who used them. The elevators were always overcrowded and tempers frayed as people waited. Arguments broke out and staff held angry protest meetings. The owners of the building were in a quandary because there was no space to install more elevators.

As business increased, staff became late for appointments and frustration rose. In desperation, the company brought in a consultant, who devised a simple solution. He lined the entire lobby with mirrors. Staff became so distracted looking at themselves and others that they forgot completely about their problems.

Replacing unproductive thoughts about pain can have a similar effect in reducing the negative emotions that accompany them.

---

stronger blast of distress message. On a personal level, there is no good reason to receive these amplified, distorted signals, because chronic pain performs no useful purpose.

The more effort you make to understand how you react to pain, the easier it is to learn how to turn the pain volume down and generally feel better.

There are two important reasons why some people suffer more pain than others. First, their volume control is permanently turned high because they are expecting pain. If you have been in daily pain for, say, 20 years, then it is understandable that you wake up in the morning waiting for it to happen. Second, the psychological factors that turn up the pain volume are part of an individual's makeup.

People who keep their pain volume turned down receive only weak signals. Listening out for warning calls does not greatly occupy their attention. They are not on alert, straining for the first indication of trouble, but more than likely are preoccupied in thinking about or doing other things. After a while, they do not even pick up some of the messages being transmitted.

Those who have acquired the knack of turning down their pain volume are basically no different from others who feel more pain. The only thing that sets them apart is their attitude. As they have discovered more about themselves and what makes them tick psychologically, their outlook on pain has become more realistic.

If, however, you have become a pain watcher and you focus your attention on pain all the time, allowing it to dominate your life – you wake in the morning and check immediately for pain; you stop working, stop mixing with people, spend all your time visiting doctors or searching for someone to help you with your pain – then it will become worse, as the psychological volume is turned up. Once you find ways of allocating less importance to pain – keeping your mind on other things, taking up interests, mixing socially and becoming active – then pain messages will inevitably become weaker and weaker.

Controlling Thinking

Problems arise when you become so preoccupied with pain that it distorts your thinking. Your perception of pain becomes unrealistic. All kinds of worries stream through your mind – the pain is much more serious than people imagine, your doctor has overlooked or misunderstood your condition, your health is probably much worse than you have been led to believe. Thoughts like these lead to *catastrophizing* – fanning the flames with exaggerated anxieties and fears. And negative thoughts nurture negative emotions, which in turn lead to negative behavior.

When you suffer chronic pain, particularly if you have had it for many years, it is important to work toward a cooler, more rational understanding of your condition, placing your pain more firmly in perspective. The way you address your pain and cope with it stems from how you address yourself. Psychologists call negative internal conversations *cognitive distortions*.

The suffering that you attribute to your pain is, in fact, the result of a number of factors. Two of the most important are:
• distress about the effects pain has on your life and daily activities;
• worries about its meaning and implications.

Your thoughts are not just a running commentary on everything you see, hear and feel. They can be an active ingredient contributing to worry and unhappiness. Past experiences, beliefs and assumptions all jostle to take over the driver's seat when your thoughts run away with you.

If, for example, you secretly believe that your pain is caused by a serious disease that no one has detected, then you may quickly imagine it becoming worse, visualize a bleak future, brood on how neglected you feel or how angry you are about the doctors who supposedly overlooked it. It isn't difficult to imagine what that does to your pain gates!

Thoughts such as these can lower your mood and make you feel hopeless about coping with pain, even make you determined to find a doctor who will do something drastic to take it all away, but none of them will help. Pat, a 44-year-old housewife, later looked back on the confusion into which pain had plunged her: "I imagined I had every disease under the sun," she said. "I was convinced everyone was hiding the awful truth from me."

Runaway thoughts, or cognitive distortions, stem from an unrealistic picture of your problems. They are not part of your imagination, but ways of thinking and describing things too harshly to yourself and not taking a balanced view. Given the opportunity, underlying beliefs can interpret almost anything as basically bad. For example, "Is this book trying to say that I don't even think right? I really must be in a hopeless mess." By studying yourself you can learn to test these thoughts against what is really happening and change them. Worry is usually about dwelling on a threat that is not present, not important and often something you can learn to cope with.

How Not to Think

Here are some ways of thinking that psychologists say lead to unnecessary worry and anxiety.

Paying selective attention to possible threatening signs, rather than giving your attention to more harmless indicators. For example, worrying that the doctor has asked for another X-ray, rather than accepting his reassurance that the investigation has been satisfactory so far.

Interpreting ambiguous signs as threatening. Deciding, for instance, that feeling weak must mean that something is wrong with your nervous system, rather than being caused by under-using your muscles.

Selectively recalling dangerous possibilities and events, which leads to overestimating the likelihood of their occurring. Reading a chest pain as a possible heart attack rather than, say, indigestion.

Anticipating negative outcomes and looking for ways of

Selective attention in operation

A nine-year-old boy came around from the anesthetic after having his appendix removed. As he lay in the recovery room with his hands over the bedclothes, the surgeon asked how he felt. The boy was relaxed and replied that he felt fine. When the surgeon left the room, the nurse asked the boy if he was worried about anything. At this point he began to cry and confessed that he was afraid of having his appendix removed. When the nurse assured him that the operation was over, he checked by slipping his hands beneath the bedclothes to feel his bandage. As soon as he realized what had happened, he immediately began to complain of pain.

escape. For example, "If I go to the movies, my back is sure to hurt. People will notice and think I'm fussing. It will spoil the evening for my friends, so I may as well not go."

Catastrophizing, or making a disaster out of a problem. "It's hurting again.... I'm no better after all this treatment.... There must be something really wrong for it to hurt so much.... All this effort is for nothing.... I don't know how I can get home with all this pain.... I'm going to crack up if this doesn't stop.... I'll have to go home for my painkillers."

Overgeneralizing. You give up in the middle of a task, thinking, "I never manage to finish anything."

Reasoning emotionally – taking your emotions as evidence. For example, "I feel hopeless about my pain getting better, so there can't be anything that will help me."

Using all-or-nothing thinking that channels your abilities in a negative direction. "I didn't manage my goal of five minutes on the exercise bike on Monday – it's obviously useless bothering to exercise at all."

Using selective abstraction – when only the negative sides of a situation are taken in and remembered. Positive ones are discounted or forgotten, especially after you achieve an important target. "Okay, I got to the supermarket and did the shopping, but I managed it only because it wasn't crowded. It took me a long time and my back hurt at the end of it. I can't just go anytime the way I used to."

Making arbitrary inferences – another way of referring to the way you interpret things to reinforce your negative self-image. For example, "The only reason people are nice to me is that they feel sorry for me because I'm obviously such a failure."

Distortions such as these make it harder to manage pain. Getting life back into perspective helps you not only to plan and succeed, but to enjoy the success you have earned.

Replace Negative Thoughts with Coping Thoughts

When you begin to study yourself, these negative thoughts can be changed by interrupting them and developing positive alternatives: "I can cope...I'm uncomfortable here, but I can control it...I'll be all right if I keep breathing and walk steadily. I've handled it without panicking – that shows I can do it better. Now I've dealt with a few bad times it should be easier.... If I go to the movies I'd better sit at the end of the row. Then if my back hurts I can get up and stand at the back for a bit, maybe do a few stretches that will help, then sit down again – my friends won't be bothered by that."

There is a different tone to these statements. They are all positive, but refer to coping with challenge or difficulty, rather than mastering it. Experience and research have shown that acknowledging the problem is more effective than trying to completely ignore it.

A mastery statement would be: *"The pain is no problem. I can work as well as I ever could."*

A coping statement would sound like: *"Although the pain makes it harder to work, I feel better if I keep going at a steady rate."*

The message here is that mastery statements set you up to fail and are not a realistic way to cope with pain, whereas coping statements are more positive and can be proved right. A patient called Pat ended his goodbye speech at his pain clinic with the words *"I am now very hopeful that, although I may still have my pain, I am going to have a better quality of life and try to enjoy it to the full."* Everyone felt that Pat's realistic attitude to coping would help him to make good progress in overcoming his pain.

Confidence plays a central part in managing your pain. It is about realistic evaluations of situations and the resources with which you face them. If you overestimate the difficulty of a situation or underestimate your ability to manage it, you diminish your chances of coping in a satisfactory way. However, when you prepare for difficulty and free yourself of failure thoughts and panic thoughts, you are much more likely to succeed. If success does not come immediately, do not feel daunted. You will be in a better position to analyze and learn from your efforts and build a base from which to move forward, working systematically toward success.

Feelings Make a Difference

Feelings are just as important as thoughts in determining how much pain you experience. Once pain dominates your thoughts and actions, it can quickly make you unhappy and depressed. You come to feel socially isolated from other people, with pain acting almost as an invisible barrier between you and the rest of the world.

It may make you feel irritable and difficult to live with, or guilty and upset because you can no longer do the things you used to do. Relationships within the family may become more difficult and strained. It may lead you to give up work, causing financial problems that make things worse. You may feel useless and become more and more dependent on other people. As you do less and less for yourself, you may become gradually more and more ruled by pain. As you feel less in control, these emotional factors add to existing problems caused by the pain.

Fear increases pain

A family physician described a woman patient who developed severe chest pains on discovering a small lump in her breast. The lump was found to be harmless, and when she was reassured, the pain subsided. Extreme emotions such as fear and anxiety can heighten the experience of pain, while the power of suggestion has the ability to lower the volume control.

The Power of Suggestion

In the 1950s, an American research team made an interesting discovery. They studied a group of patients with severe pain who were going to be treated with morphine. Without explaining the experiment, they replaced the drug with an inactive sugar pill (a placebo) and found that about 35 percent of those patients reported a marked improvement in their pain. The figure was particularly remarkable since morphine itself is effective in only about 75 percent of cases. Staff caring for the patients did not know whether they were administering morphine or a placebo. They were, however, very encouraging and optimistic, instilling a positive attitude in their patients. Reducing people's anxiety and thinking positively in this way, without the use of active drugs, proved extremely effective. A few years

Measuring pain

Measuring pain is not an easy business because of its subjective nature, nor is it a good idea for an individual to become too preoccupied with charting and recording it. However, if you are working on ways of reducing your pain levels, it is sometimes useful to record what progress you have made. There is a simple method for keeping a rough track of how your pain changes, known as the Visual Analogue Scale. This, it should be said, is a very personal indicator and not a method of comparing one person's pain with another.

Take a piece of paper and draw a horizontal line about 4 inches (10 cm) long. A "round-number" measurement is ideal so that you can calibrate the line with a ruler to keep a more accurate record. One end of the line represents no pain at all, while the other indicates the worst possible pain you can imagine:

NO PAIN |————————————————————| WORST PAIN EVER

If you mark the line every day at a point that you think corresponds to the amount of pain you are suffering, and measure it with a ruler, you can keep track of how your pain changes on different days according to how you are working to reduce it.

earlier, a similar experiment had been carried out on patients suffering from severe headaches, resulting in 52 percent reporting noticeable improvement.

The power of suggestion is also reflected in the success rate of hypnosis in pain treatment. The ability to change your outlook and attitude is a key to achieving positive results. Trying to cope with emotional aspects of pain means trying to change what you think and do in response to pain. One of the important starting points is not to think about pain, or dwell on it, any more than is necessary. The more you can divert your mind into other interests and activities, the more you will find it possible to distract yourself from pain and the less intense it will feel. Most of us have experienced a small injury or cut that only began to hurt when we noticed it. Some people are able to train their minds to almost switch off pain by relaxing or concentrating their thoughts in certain ways.

McGill–Melzack Pain Questionnaire

So how do you know how well you are coping with pain?

We know that how we cope depends on whether the pain volume is turned up or down by thoughts, feelings and what we do. One way of gauging our inner state is by taking note of how we express thoughts and emotions in terms of language.

Pain is a country of the mind and, like any country, has its own language. Ronald Melzack, a professor of psychology at McGill University in Montreal, devised a questionnaire that is used internationally for measuring pain more accurately. You can use it yourself to obtain a general indication of how well you are coping.

The McGill–Melzack Pain Questionnaire contains groups of words that each describe a particular type of pain. People are asked to choose the word in each group that best describes the way they feel. If the words in one or more groups do not fit the pain, the person does not select any in that group or groups. Only those that completely match what the person is suffering are chosen.

You are using the questionnaire here for a slightly different purpose, but the method of picking the word group most appropriate to you is the same.

Fill in this questionnaire now, concerning your pain, before reading on:

McGill–Melzack Pain Questionnaire

Look carefully at the 20 groups of words. *If* any word in the group applies to *your* pain, please circle that word – but *do not circle more than one word in any one group*. If more than one word in a group applies to your pain, you should circle *only the most suitable word* in that group. In groups that *do not apply* to your pain, there is no need to circle any word – just leave them unmarked.

1
Flickering
Quivering
Pulsing
Throbbing
Beating
Pounding

2
Jumping
Flashing
Shooting

3
Pricking
Boring
Drilling
Stabbing
Lancinating

4
Sharp
Cutting
Lacerating

5
Pinching
Pressing
Gnawing
Cramping
Crushing

6
Tugging
Pulling
Wrenching

7
Hot
Burning
Scalding
Searing

8
Tingling
Itchy
Smarting
Stinging

9
Dull
Sore
Hurting
Aching
Heavy

10
Tender
Taut
Rasping
Splitting

11
Tiring
Exhausting

12
Sickening
Suffocating

13
Fearful
Frightful
Terrifying

14
Punishing
Grueling
Cruel
Vicious
Killing

15
Wretched
Binding

16
Annoying
Troublesome
Miserable
Intense
Unbearable

17
Spreading
Radiating
Penetrating
Piercing

18
Tight
Numb
Drawing
Squeezing
Tearing

19
Cool
Cold
Freezing

20
Nagging
Nauseating
Agonizing
Dreadful
Torturing

The McGill–Melzack Pain Questionnaire recognizes that pain consists of different dimensions. Answers indicate both the sensory and the emotional aspects of pain, which vary in different people at different times. Pain sufferers use words that show how much emotional distress is associated with their problem. If, for example, you ask some people what their pain is like, they may say, "It's horrible," or "It's miserable," "It's wearing, depressing, frustrating," or "It gets me down." These are all terms that describe the effects of pain, rather than the pain itself.

Other people might choose words that describe the sensory aspects of pain: "It's a sharp pain," "A stabbing pain," "A tingling pain," "A hot, burning pain." If you study the language, or vocabulary, of pain carefully there are clues to which aspect you are talking about. The word groups you have chosen give an insight into how much pain has begun to dominate your life in terms of psychological distress. Generally, when you are coping well with your pain you are aware of its physical sensation but do not feel that it is controlling your life. You feel on top of it and are not threatened, miserable or depressed. When you describe your pain, it is in terms of how it feels physically.

If you are not managing to cope too well, the pain is overbearing and you feel worn down. It depresses you and you tend to use emotional words to describe it. The word groups you have chosen are a broad indicator of the psychological balance you are managing to achieve.

The farther down the group you go, the more relevant it becomes to the interpretation of your pain. That is, if you circle the first word in a group, it is not as significant as if you circle the middle word, and this in turn is not as significant as if you circle the last word.

Human beings, of course, are not always so straightforward and compartmentalized. Some people may describe a stabbing, shooting pain in physical terms, but still feel that it has taken over their lives. A rule of thumb is that if you can accept your pain and come to terms with it, then it is likely to be physical pain. If you find it unbearable, then the time has come to examine the psychological causes. If you do not, then the pain is unlikely to improve.

Look particularly at word groups 11, 12, 13, 14, 15, 16 and 20. If you have circled these more than any others, pain is causing you psychological distress that you need to address. The farther down these word groups you go, the worse your psychological distress is. Thus, if the pain is "terrifying," "killing" and "unbearable" rather than "fearful" and "annoying," or "torturing" rather than "nagging," this indicates more distress.

While the Visual Analogue Scale provides a sum total for your whole experience of pain, the McGill–Melzack Pain Questionnaire gives a deeper indication of how much mental distress it is causing. To discover more about yourself in relation to your problems, there are more questions you can answer. Questionnaires are a good way to guide you through this because pain often alters the way you look at things.

Pain and Depression Are Linked

It is common for people suffering long-term pain to become depressed and, conversely, for patients suffering depression to experience aches and pains they would not normally have. This is because there is a link between pain and depression that is important to understand.

Depression is not an isolated feeling but something that may take the form of a physical experience. Chemicals released in the brain during some forms of depression are also transmitters of pain messages, which is why 60 percent of depression sufferers also experience pain of one kind or another.

A woman, for example, suffered a back pain whose origins

Pain Coping Indicator

When pain distorts your ability to reason clearly it is not easy to observe yourself in a detached way. Dr. Eric Ghadiali, a neuropsychologist, devised a questionnaire that helps to overcome this problem. Circle the appropriate word to indicate how much you agree or disagree with the following statements. It is important to answer all the questions.

1. I feel happy about my life in general.
   strongly disagree   disagree   uncertain   agree   agree strongly

2. I have lost my confidence.
   strongly disagree   disagree   uncertain   agree   agree strongly

3. I try to avoid other people when I have pain.
   strongly disagree   disagree   uncertain   agree   agree strongly

4. I feel my pain cuts me off from other people.
   strongly disagree   disagree   uncertain   agree   agree strongly

5. I sometimes worry that I have a serious illness.
   strongly disagree   disagree   uncertain   agree   agree strongly

6. My pain affects the way I get on with family and friends a great deal.
   strongly disagree   disagree   uncertain   agree   agree strongly

7. My pain makes me feel tense and frustrated.
   strongly disagree   disagree   uncertain   agree   agree strongly

8. My pain makes me feel miserable most of the time.
   strongly disagree   disagree   uncertain   agree   agree strongly

9. I have to rely on other people a great deal because of my pain.
   strongly disagree   disagree   uncertain   agree   agree strongly

10. I never go out because people do not want to know you when you have pain.
    strongly disagree   disagree   uncertain   agree   agree strongly

11. My pain stops me from leading a normal life.
    strongly disagree   disagree   uncertain   agree   agree strongly

12. I find it very difficult to relax.
    strongly disagree   disagree   uncertain   agree   agree strongly

13. My pain makes me opt out of things.
    strongly disagree   disagree   uncertain   agree   agree strongly

14. My pain stops me going places.
    strongly disagree   disagree   uncertain   agree   agree strongly

15. My pain makes it difficult to socialize with people.
    strongly disagree   disagree   uncertain   agree   agree strongly

16. I am coping well with my pain.
    strongly disagree   disagree   uncertain   agree   agree strongly

17. My pain makes me feel useless and not needed.
    strongly disagree   disagree   uncertain   agree   agree strongly

18. All my problems are caused by pain.
    strongly disagree   disagree   uncertain   agree   agree strongly

19. I manage to do most things in my life that I want to do.
    strongly disagree   disagree   uncertain   agree   agree strongly

Now see how you fared. Questions 1, 16 and 19 score: strongly disagree, 1; disagree, 2; uncertain, 3; agree, 4; strongly agree, 5. All other questions score: strongly disagree, 5; disagree, 4; uncertain, 3; agree, 2; strongly agree, 1.

Most people with long-standing pain problems achieve somewhere around 50 on this test. If your score is above 65, then you are probably coping quite well with your pain and not allowing it to interfere with your life a great deal. The higher the score, the better you are at managing your life.

A score below 40 means that you are very likely having difficulty living a normal life. You may feel a loss of confidence and have perhaps stopped mixing with people. Basically, you do not feel very happy with yourself and possibly feel that pain is controlling you. It is likely that you need some help in improving your coping skills.

The longer you have pain, the more likely it is you will feel depressed. Even in normal circumstances people tend to brood over their problems when they feel under the weather. Pain magnifies black moods, making it harder to change your habits and behavior.

You have probably gathered by now how difficult it is to quantify pain, because what you are trying to measure is a personal experience that, quite often, you believe no one else fully understands. Even when the pain is all psychological, however, and there are no obvious physical symptoms, it is no less real.

could not be pinpointed until she began to talk about her life. It emerged that her husband had lost his job and they had no money to pay their rent. Their domestic situation had brought on depression that resulted in pain. Her case proved particularly easy to address. When government benefits were arranged to ease their financial situation, the pain cleared up.

Broadly, there are two kinds of depression. *Reactive* depression is experienced when your house is uninsured and burns down, the family walk out and, on top of everything, the budgie dies. The most common cause of depression in people with chronic pain is a reaction to their pain and what is happening to them as they lose control of their lives. However, like the chicken and the egg, it is important to realize that in some people the problem starts off with depression, which causes the pain.

Endogenous depression, which means growing from within as opposed to reacting to outside circumstances, is the result of biochemical changes within the brain and is a medical condition. The sufferer may have a successful career, a loving family and a wonderful future, but still feels terribly, inexplicably depressed.

As with pain, it would be futile to say that depression is imagined. Obviously, the person who is so miserable actually feels miserable and no doctor would suggest otherwise. In the same way, it is futile to say that someone who feels in pain is not feeling it, even if the cause might be psychological, in particular depression.

Depression is one of the most common psychological difficulties that turn up the volume control of pain. The link between pain and depression makes chronic-pain sufferers feel cut off from other people and unable to do things they used to do. They often lose their confidence and feel a sense of diminished control. As they become more and more isolated, their world becomes increasingly dominated by pain, and their depression increases.

Fight Depression with Activity
If you feel yourself coming down or sliding into a trough of

depression, the most effective way to get through it is to activate yourself. Generally, when you try to head off a bout of depression or lift yourself from it, anything you can do that gives you a sense of regaining control of your life is therapeutic. It may be a regular exercise or relaxation program, or even something as small as doing a crossword or reading a book. The aim is to achieve an element of success and to experience the feeling of being in control again.

Chronic pain is an isolating experience and it is easy to feel quite cut off and alone. There is always benefit in mixing with other people as much as possible and keeping active, which is why relaxation groups, yoga classes and tai chi sessions can be particularly helpful.

Other Psychological Factors Affecting Pain

There are other manifestations of psychological pain that are more extreme and less commonly encountered. In some patients, for example, phobias may be expressed in terms of very real pain. In cases of delusion, patients often continue to suffer pain whatever treatments are administered.

Perfectionism, which is a kind of obsession, is another psychological dimension of pain. No matter how low patients of this type manage to turn down the pain volume, they are never satisfied that it is enough. Only a complete absence of pain will meet the exacting demands they place on themselves.

This is another example of unreasonable ideals that work against overcoming pain. If these people have pain that is of quite a low level, say 1 out of 10, they are often unable to cope because their perfectionism stops them from accepting any pain at all. Consequently, they will amplify their pain intensity several times over because they are deeply unhappy. More easygoing individuals would possibly not even notice a pain level so low.

When No Physical Cause for Pain Exists

There are also patients who, for many reasons, have excruciating pain for which no physical cause can be traced. The treatment is often unorthodox, but underlines the importance of understanding the psychological background to each individual problem.

Some patients in a pain clinic were talking about work one day, when a woman jokingly referred to her supervisor as a pain in the neck. Everyone laughed until someone remarked that the patient's problem was, in fact, a pain in the neck. She had been told by her doctor that she had arthritis in her spine, but an examination had indicated that there was not sufficient arthritis to justify this as the cause of the pain. When she was questioned further about work, she recalled that her pain had briefly cleared up the week her supervisor had been on holiday. When the patient herself was on holiday the pain also improved, which led her to believe that rest had a beneficial effect. "Work makes it worse," she remarked, then realized for the first time that it was not her job, but her supervisor, with whom there was often friction, that caused her pain. The patient changed her job and took up similar work in another factory. She still had a little pain, but was able to function quite happily. It was a case of a boss quite literally being a pain in the neck.

Another woman had suffered from a pain in her leg for five years for which her doctor and staff could find no explanation. They knew that she was widowed but had no idea of the cause of her psychological pain until she spoke of her husband's death. He had been hit by a car and taken to an intensive care unit, where doctors decided that his badly crushed leg would have to be amputated. His wife, who thought his leg was simply broken, was shocked when she was told that the leg had had to be removed. Shortly afterward, her husband died.

As she talked more about the traumatic experience, she recalled that her pain had begun as she walked out of hospital after hearing about her husband's emergency operation. The pain was in her left leg, and her husband had had his left leg amputated. It was felt that this was the reason she was in chronic pain, but she refused to accept it and continued to insist that the cause was physical and no doctor had been able to diagnose it. The woman was last heard of still seeking a cure. The staff had found to their satisfaction what had caused the pain, but, sadly, the conclusion was not to the patient's satisfaction.

Another patient had a burning facial pain. Nothing physically wrong could be found, though there was no doubt that she was genuinely suffering. The pain was eventually traced back to when she was 16 and intervened in a fight between her father and mother. The father struck a blow at the mother, which landed on the girl's face. She ran from the house in shock to her boyfriend's, where his family took her in. The patient was too frightened to go back to her parents and married her boyfriend. Soon afterward, her mother and father divorced and then died. Her pain was associated with guilt because she had left her mother and because she had never made it up with her father before his death. After psychoanalysis her facial pain disappeared.

These are unusual cases, but they illustrate how deep-rooted psychological pain can become and how important it is to increase your understanding of yourself and develop an awareness of your thoughts, feelings and actions.

Pain Habits

When chronic pain takes hold of people's thoughts and emotions, it begins to dictate the way they behave in everyday life. Chronic-pain sufferers send out signals that they have a problem. It may be through facial expressions, rubbing their backs, limping, wearing a surgical collar or perhaps spending most of their time in a wheelchair.

It is important to ask yourself what kind of pain signals you send out. A psychological situation many long-term pain sufferers find themselves locked into is that pain makes them "special." People ask how they are feeling, help out with the shopping or strenuous work and solicitously inquire if they have had their pills. Life appears to offer a number of bonuses when they cast themselves in the role of pain victim. When they were well, they probably received only a fraction of the attention and worked hard for their family with little acknowledgment or appreciation. Domestic pets discover that if they behave in a certain way, they get a reward, and some pain sufferers have unconsciously learned similar behavior. If they send out signals of pain and suffering, people around them react in a favorable manner.

Once you condition yourself to avoid doing things because of pain, your behavior becomes a difficult habit to break. It is like someone limping to avoid pain and continuing when the injury has healed because it brought help and attention.

Behaving in a certain way to sidestep something unpleasant is similar to the little boy who banged a bass drum around the streets all day to keep the lions and tigers away.

"But there aren't any lions and tigers," someone said.

"See how well it works," he replied.

Once avoidance behavior begins, it is difficult to stop. It helps to keep the cycle of pain revolving, until, in some cases, people actually prefer being pain victims because, despite the suffering, it gives their lives a dimension previously lacking.

Break Pain Habits by Targeting

An effective method of helping yourself to break pain habits, which we touched on in chapter 3, is gradually reducing negative actions through *targeting* – setting small, achievable objectives that unlearn bad pain behavior and promote positive activity. If you sit in a wheelchair to avoid pain, or wear a collar for the same reason, you can work on a program that will gradually reduce the time you spend doing this each day.

Some people feel that pain may not have affected their lives to any great degree. If this is genuinely the case, then it is still a good idea to think about areas of your life in which you would like to see change. It can be difficult to become motivated, and we all find at times that it is easy to get into a rut and put off things that need to be done. The purpose of targeting is to consider ways of reversing the changes pain has made in your life. In order to set a target you need to take time to honestly assess what these changes are. Here are a few examples of activities that may have been curtailed by pain:

- social life – refusing invitations to visit friends, go to parties or on family outings;
- traveling in cars, buses and trains;
- driving;
- housework – certain chores may be difficult because of bending, etc.;
- gardening;
- shopping;
- sitting for long periods of time – this may, for example, affect going to the movies or the theater;
- walking distances.

Having identified an area you would like to change, you need to draw up guidelines to help you set your target. It may be that you want to pursue a particular target that will require some time to achieve. Do not let this put you off. It may be possible to take a gradual approach, increasing your activity step by step until, eventually, you have successfully achieved it.

Guidelines for targeting

1. Consider an area you really want to change or improve upon.
2. Be realistic about your target. Try not to choose a task that is initially too far beyond your capabilities. Alternatively, do not succumb to bad pain behavior and underestimate yourself.
3. Be specific so that you can measure your achievements.
4. Try not to incorporate too many variables: make sure your selection is not too dependent on other people, good weather, etc. In other words, when you make a contract with yourself, do not build in an escape clause.
5. Always be positive.
6. Consider the possibility, if you wish, of setting yourself more than one target.

Targeting is a useful way of understanding more about yourself. Pain has a way of blurring the edges of reality, so it is important to use techniques to rediscover yourself and examine why and how you may have changed with pain.

Honesty Is Best

When pain is the most important thing in your life, a meeting with your doctor can crucially affect which direction your emotions take. How you react to your doctor's comments and observations can generate feelings that, in some cases, may actually lead to your pain increasing.

Many people feel, for example, that their doctors have been rude, offhand, kept them waiting for long periods and dismissed their pain as imaginary. Many react to the way they feel they have been treated with anger and a sense of isolation, rejection and depression. Some say, "I go to my family doctor expecting success. When I don't find it, I feel lost and let down.

I don't know where to turn." They tend to be people who hoped that their doctor would take control and lift their pain from them. When she or he was unable to do so, they felt abandoned and in limbo. "I didn't know what to do," one patient recalled. "I felt I couldn't go on after that."

It was only when they discovered the pain management program that they learned that the solution lay with them. In effect, after visiting many doctors, they had become the real specialists in their own pain. No one else could experience it or know what it was like because it belonged only to them. Harboring resentment and anger toward their doctors only resulted in prolonging their pain.

Another common complaint is that visiting different doctors often achieves little more than being offered different explanations. One doctor gives one reason for their pain, while another may suggest something else entirely. These people never felt they were getting the same answer twice and were left in a state of increasing confusion.

It is possible that the doctors, perhaps sensing that these people desperately wanted an explanation, felt obliged to offer them one. It was only when these sufferers met a doctor who specialized in pain that they encountered someone with the courage to say, "I don't know why you've got this pain. I can only guess at it. How to go on from here is now the real issue."

In some cases, people cannot understand their pain because no one can. They are searching for an explanation that is somehow structured and easy to understand, something they can visualize and grasp. Having received it, the next question is "So, why can't you make me better?"

People too obsessed with the mechanism of their pain – striving to discover exactly what the reasons are for it – struggle to apply logic to something that may be impossible to understand logically. Trying to offload their problem onto a doctor and then blaming the doctor for not being able to provide a miracle is not taking full responsibility for their pain. Unless they accept responsibility, they cannot hope to regain control.

Honesty is a great asset. Many pain sufferers run such a gauntlet of symptoms, thoughts and emotions between visits to their doctor that it is difficult to keep track of how they feel and what they expect from him or her. If you experience such problems, it is better to put time aside and work out what questions you would like your doctor to answer. Write them down. On your next visit, explain that it is difficult in the short time available to say clearly what is on your mind, and refer to your sheet of paper.

Problems and resentment arise when people who may have a life of pain feel that they are being allocated only two minutes for what is the most important thing in the world to them.

Speaking your mind clearly, without the distraction of negative feelings, often requires a little assertiveness. Business people frequently use assertiveness in their training. It is not aggression, but a tactful, honest and straightforward way of informing people of what you want. Assertiveness is a useful asset for regaining control over your life. It may mean choosing not to speak out or, on occasion, choosing to lose an argument. It may mean admitting mistakes, being gentle and tactful and allowing other people to be assertive too.

Thinking carefully about what you say and expressing yourself honestly and diplomatically should not offend people. If it does, then that is their problem, not yours. Making efforts to be more assertive will develop your confidence, help you to take control of your emotions and regain control of your own situation.

Trying to understand more about yourself and studying how your thoughts, feeling and actions relate to pain will help you cope more effectively.

Golden rules for managing pain

- Try not to let pain dominate what you do or what you think about. Try not to dwell on pain or think about it too much. It helps if you can distract yourself by keeping busy and interested in as many other things as possible.
- Try not to avoid doing things because of your pain. Don't use your pain as an excuse not to do something – even to yourself. Try to keep control of what you do and not allow pain to dominate your life.
- Try not to talk about your pain. Try to look as fit and healthy as possible. Never make a show of being in pain, either by talking about it or by actions that may signal others that you have a pain problem.
- Try not to be too negative. Try to always think about positive aspects of your life and concentrate on good things that are happening.
- Don't look for miracle cures. They very rarely happen, and while you are waiting, things usually get much worse.
- Take control of yourself. Learn relaxation techniques, exercise regularly and keep yourself as mentally and physically active as you can. Keep up your interests and relationships with other people. When you increase your activities, do so gradually. Don't try to do too much too soon.

SEVEN

Pain and Other People

Everyone thrives on attention – without it we would suffer from emotional starvation. Pain sufferers generally send out more signals for attention than do family, friends and colleagues who do not have the same health problems. Because your pain demands attention from you, in turn your behavior demands attention from others. It may be through a pained expression, a gesture indicating suffering, a groan, a tone of voice, a wince or a dozen other ways that you transmit to the world that all is not well.

Pain is the cuckoo in the nest of normal living. As it occupies your time, it grows bigger, demanding more and more, until feelings of happiness, confidence and self-esteem are elbowed out. Your subconscious, like an anxious mother bird, constantly reminds you that the monster that has taken over requires increasing time and attention.

Broadcasting Your Pain Is Self-Defeating

Pain has a voracious appetite for attention. No matter how much time you devote to pain, it usually demands more.

Without realizing it, you may be constantly sending out signals for sympathy and attention. It is similar to screech behavior in babies, which we touched on in chapter 3. The baby learns that if it screams it will be picked up. When the harassed mother tries not to pick it up, it screams louder. In the same way, pain sufferers may subconsciously turn up the volume control of their pain to gain attention from family and friends. Unfortunately, in the process they increase and prolong their own suffering.

If, for example, you complain of a headache, your partner may be very understanding and offer to do the dishes. If you complain again after dinner the following evening, he or she may be a little less sympathetic. After a week of this behavior, you will almost certainly be guaranteed little sympathy. To obtain the attention you received on day one, you would by now probably have to writhe on the floor, clutching your head.

To achieve the level of attention your pain demands, you have to increase your suffering. Your subconscious, desperately needing a reaction of sympathy, tenderness, concern, support or help, turns up the pain volume by opening your pain gates to obtain the response it previously acquired with only a small amount of pain.

If you are in chronic pain, it is important to ask yourself if your family and friends tend to take notice only when you cast yourself in the role of a pain victim.

When you send out pain signals, there are usually two ways in which those around you react – both of them wrong. They are either unsympathetic and ignore you, starving you of attention and refusing to believe you are in pain; or, possibly worse, they become overattentive, doing jobs for you and offering help at every opportunity. They force you to adopt the role of an invalid.

When this kind of suffocating behavior is prolonged it can

sometimes turn relatives into dynamic seekers after a cure. They wheel their partner from doctor to doctor and speak completely on his or her behalf. The patient becomes a glove puppet, almost an inanimate object, while the husband or wife who does not have the pain takes over the show.

This kind of reaction is demeaning to pain sufferers; it removes their dignity, confidence and self-respect. It is easy to be judgmental about relatives who act this way, but there is every possibility that the patient has encouraged much of it by sending out "helpless" signals. Families of pain sufferers have to walk a fine line. A delicate balance exists between ignoring people in chronic pain and trying to do too much for them. Starving them of attention is as unkind as suffocating them with it.

The fact that people broadcast their pain really means that their subconscious is trying to attract attention or divert them from exercise, relaxation or whatever efforts they are making to overcome pain. The more determined they are to take positive steps and conquer their disability, the louder their subconscious screams that they are pain patients and deserve some attention.

Treat people as ill and they become ill

Some mischievous medical students decided to play a joke on a particularly obnoxious colleague. When he came into the lounge, they remarked that he looked quite pale and asked if he felt all right. The student protested that he had never felt better. Then more students walked in and made similar comments. This went on until, by the end of the afternoon, the student had convinced himself that he was ill and, amid great hilarity, slipped out to the emergency room for a checkup.

The same principle worked for African witch doctors, who could kill people because everyone believed they had the power to do it. If the witch doctor told people that they were going to die, then generally they would. This does not work in our society because we are not conditioned to believe it. However, it is possible to make people feel ill simply by the way you treat them.

How to treat a family member in chronic pain

If a member of your family is in chronic pain, here are three useful guidelines:

1. Encourage your relative to be as active as possible. Don't talk about or dwell on the pain too much. Try not to overdo the sympathy. Don't keep asking, for example, "How's the pain today?" or "How are you feeling?" This only reminds your relative that he or she has pain, and it will probably make things worse.
2. Encourage your relative to be as independent as possible. Try not to do too much for him or her.
3. If your relative dwells on pain and talks about it constantly, try to change the subject or distract him or her with something more interesting. Encourage your relative to exercise, to learn relaxation skills, to take up interests and to think about more positive aspects of life.

The cues, as we've said, may be verbal, in the form of groans, sighs, "ouches" and complaints; or visual, such as limping, restless movements, tortured facial expressions or rubbing the painful area. The need for attention may be expressed in agitated, tense, depressed or withdrawn behavior, or in using equipment such as collars, braces, slings, canes, wheelchairs and gadgets.

Groaning, limping or withdrawing into yourself does not help the pain, but is simply a form of communication to tell people you are in distress. It may be considered unkind to make similar comments about surgical appliances, but there is no scientific evidence to suggest that many of these devices are more than psychological props. To wear them for a few weeks is fine, but people who have been walking around for two years in a brace or collar display it as a badge to announce that they are disabled. It is almost medically impossible to support the neck or spine by means of a brace or collar. Both tend to make the muscles stiff and tense, and when they are removed after prolonged use, the muscles are by then too weak to support the affected area. The patient has to put the collar, for example, back on to help do the work the muscles have become unable to perform.

Sending Positive Messages Makes a Difference

Sufferers who make pain faces or clutch at themselves are not helping their pain, and this is really just a signal that their pain is fighting to retain its hold on their subconscious. People who persist in being positive can pass through this barrier and firmly establish who is in charge. It is important to recognize that your pain, and the way it makes you feel and act, has a significant effect on others. If you send out messages that you are in pain, people will treat you as an invalid, not an individual. The way they treat you will in turn determine how well you cope. Whether you complain that you hurt and can't do anything, or simply send out nonverbal messages, it amounts to the same thing. People respond to what you broadcast.

If, for example, someone asks how you are and you reply, "Terrible," the scene for the conversation is immediately set. The person feels wary and a little nervous because you are not feeling well. Someone who replies, "Great," or "Wonderful," puts the other person at ease. The conversation, from this point, is more likely to go up than down. It is surprising that saying "Great," even when you don't feel it, not only helps the other person but actually lifts the conversation, so that by the end you actually feel good yourself.

There are times, of course, when it is important to confide in someone about how you feel, but only in the right situation. It is much better to develop a habit of being positive than to gain a reputation for moaning.

One patient, David, sustained multiple fractures when a car hit him, throwing him across the road. He walked heavily stooped and with a cane. He had remained at work but found office life difficult to cope with. His biggest complaint was, "If only people would treat me normally. They regard me as a cripple. I never get asked to do ordinary things anymore, such as making coffee. It's very demeaning." When David was asked how people knew he was disabled, he said he supposed that it was because he used a cane and kept it handy on his desk. It was suggested that if he could manage without it, it might be better to leave it in his car. He tried this and wrote several weeks later: "I feel great. Yesterday, someone in the office said, 'Come on, David, it's your turn to make coffee. Don't think you can get out of it.' They accepted me as normal. And because they made me feel normal, it is now much easier to cope."

It is important to become aware of pain signals, make every effort to reduce them to a minimum and persuade your family and friends to treat you normally. Look as fit and healthy as you possibly can. Rather than discuss what you are unable to do or how much pain you have, talk about what you can do and the targets you have achieved. It is more positive to talk about the five minutes you have spent walking than the 12 hours you have spent lying in bed.

Success depends on families working together, but this is not always easy. One patient, Doris, suffered from a bad back and had difficulty standing or lifting. She was the center of her family and worked hard looking after her husband and three grown-up sons. Her ambition was to return home and cook the Sunday lunch.

Doris set herself targets, breaking them down to work on all the aspects of cooking a meal: standing for an hour, lifting weights comparable to a full saucepan, bending to put things into the oven. The meal was a great success, but the event turned into a disaster. When her family finished Sunday lunch, they went out for a walk, leaving Doris with the cleanup, which she found difficult to cope with. They'd assumed that because she had cooked a meal, she was better. They should have invited her to join them or, if she found the walk too difficult, offered to stay at home to keep her company. Instead, they ignored her. Doris had to explain that they needed to be more supportive and that her big day had turned out to be a disappointment.

Chronic pain inevitably affects your relationships with family, friends and colleagues. The wrong kind of pain behavior occurs when pain has eroded your confidence and sense of self-worth. The position pain forces you into and the resulting demands you place on people around you diminish your self-esteem and desire to succeed.

Actions and feelings relating to pain are closely linked. It is difficult, for example, to slump in a chair with your shoulders hunched and say, "I feel great." Somehow, it lacks conviction. Equally, it feels odd to throw back your shoulders, stick out your chest, punch the air and shout, "I feel depressed." How you act sends signals inwardly to yourself as well as outwardly to others.

Body Talk

Body language – the visual signals your body is sending out – has a profound effect on both yourself and others. Even sitting

---

The Sarnoff Squeeze

There are times when even high-flying professionals feel anxiety and a loss of control in stressful situations. This is a familiar situation to many chronic-pain sufferers. Professional public speakers use a way of calming themselves and regaining control, called the Sarnoff Squeeze.

The method is to squeeze the palms of your hands together while breathing in. The deeper you inhale, the more tightly you squeeze your hands together. When your lungs are full, exhale slowly while releasing the pressure on your palms. Anxiety ebbs, replaced by a feeling of calmness and control. If the exercise is too conspicuous to do when other people are around, you can achieve the same results by pressing your palms against the arms of a chair.

in the right position affects your mind and how you feel about yourself. When you feel "down" and sink into yourself there is no room for your diaphragm to move and you take the kind of small, shallow breaths associated with depression. Sitting straight, getting yourself and your spirits as high as possible, improves the way you feel.

Getting Comfortable with Your Body

People with chronic pain are often unhappy with their bodies. As pain progresses, making life miserable, they sometimes develop resentment against the particular part that gives them problems. This is not unusual, since most of us have some aspect of our bodies we wish could be more perfect. Pain merely exaggerates this feeling in a negative way.

Feeling comfortable about your body is part of learning to like yourself and rebuilding self-esteem. It is unreasonable to expect people to like and respect you if you don't like and respect yourself. Some people tend to live their lives as Fords wishing they were Rolls-Royces. When they are unhappy with themselves, they tend to lock themselves in a mental garage, turn off their engine and say, "I'm not going anywhere. I'm going to sit here and wait until I become a Rolls."

Pain makes people react this way; they retreat into themselves in the hope that one day everything will be all right. Like an unused car, they will probably succeed only in becoming more and more rusty, until they are unable to move.

A good example is postherpetic neuralgia, a pain that goes on intolerably after nerve damage from shingles, especially in elderly people. Many sufferers do as little as possible, thinking, "When the pain goes, I'll restart my life." They wait – and after a year find they have the same amount of pain. They stop visiting their friends, going shopping, doing housework or seeing their family. After perhaps three or four years of this, they consult their doctor, who probably prescribes painkillers. They should realize instead that while their pain may be around for another four years, the quality of their lives is slipping away. The only advice of any practical value is, don't wait – become active again.

An Exercise to Boost Body Image

Pain patients who lose confidence because of their bodies find it difficult to maintain relationships with other people. A useful exercise, which may help, is aimed at making friends with your body again, becoming more aware of it and accepting pain without resentment.

It works like this. Take off your clothes, standing in front of a full-length mirror, and take stock of yourself. Starting at the top of your head with your hair, move down your body, making a list of all the parts that you dislike or that you consider are less than perfect. You may wish for your hair to be curly instead of straight, your ears to be smaller, your nose bigger and so on. Be as objective as possible, as though the body you are looking at belongs to someone else. As you travel down, concentrate too on the parts you are happy with, feeling pleased that you are comfortable with them.

When you have studied yourself right down to your toes, place a hand on the first part of your body you felt unhappy with. Say, "I'm sorry for criticizing you and disliking you. You've been a good (arm, leg, stomach, etc.) You've done your best over the years. You're not perfect, but you're part of me. I haven't been able to function properly because of you, but I love you."

At first, you may feel self-conscious doing this exercise, but it is a private dialogue between you and your body. It concerns no one else and is an effective way of being kinder to yourself. Many people come to terms with themselves and feel more at ease after doing this exercise.

Building Confidence and Self-Esteem

If you are in pain you need to feel good about yourself and the environment you find yourself in, even if it is not positive or supportive. You can never get a guarantee that wherever you go, whether to the local drugstore or an interview for a job, people are going to be kind and understanding. Self-confidence and self-esteem are built by feeling good about yourself even when people may not be feeling good toward you. The aim is not to be reliant on others for the way you feel about yourself. If you are in chronic pain, what you transmit is possibly negative and what you send out governs the messages you are going to receive back and how they affect you.

When you are in pain your subconscious constantly urges you to play safe. This, as we know, is not wise advice. When you look back on your life, all the major decisions you have made have been based on risk. Taking exams, your first date, getting married – all carried a risk of failure, but also an overriding hope that they would work out. Changing your life always involves risk, but change is difficult if you lack confidence. Life, in this respect, is a little like playing poker. You may not have a good hand, but if you appear confident, you increase your chances of winning. Confidence and self-esteem go hand in hand to improve your image of yourself and your relationships with others. They enable you to go for a job interview, or be in a situation that perhaps does not work out, and carry on.

Eliminate Avoidance Behavior

The first step in building these positive aspects to help you overcome pain is to make an all-out effort to eliminate negative pain behavior. One important question to ask yourself: Do you ever use your pain as an excuse to get out of doing something? If you do, there may be other issues to sort out in your life before you can go forward and take on your main objective of conquering pain.

Pain is like a balance sheet. On one side, there occasionally appear to be benefits – pain gets you attention; it helps you avoid doing things you don't enjoy; at times there are even financial compensations. But there is a debit side. Once you try to use pain to your advantage, it always comes back to trap you in a worse situation.

Sometimes, it helps to be more honest with yourself and ask what lies behind your reasons for acting and thinking a certain way. One patient, Neville Shone, made this voyage of self-discovery and went on to write an excellent book about his experiences (see Further Resources). He had had a benign tumor removed from his spine, and although the operation was successful, his spinal cord was partially damaged, leaving him with chronic back pain.

When Neville's wife asked him to help her with the Saturday shopping, he complained that his back was hurting and used the pain as an excuse to get out of something he did not enjoy. Instead, he spent the afternoon pleasantly watching TV. Then Neville realized that he had to accept that his pain also prevented him from driving into town to visit his friends and from attending a football game in the afternoon. By turning up his pain volume to avoid shopping, he had also missed the activities he really enjoyed.

Neville thought about his actions more carefully and decided to take another approach. What he should have said, he realized, was something like "I've got back pain and I don't particularly enjoy shopping. I don't want to make it worse doing something I don't find much fun. If you can manage the shopping, I'll have a rest and we could go to the movies tonight. It may make my back hurt, but at least we will have a good time together."

By accepting that he was going to have pain regardless, he opted for having pain doing something he would enjoy. His wife had no objection to shopping alone and looked forward to an evening with her husband. The decision also left him free to see his friends.

Sex and Pain

Sexual relationships are an area where pain is often used as an avoidance excuse, by men as often as women. "Not tonight, dear – I've got a headache" has become a cliché. The partner who makes the excuse may not have a massive headache, but uses it to get out of sex for another reason. Instead of saying, perhaps, "I don't want sex because your feet smell," the partner is saying, "I don't want sex because there is something wrong with me."

This is another illusionary "benefit" of pain – by telling a white lie, one partner avoids sex without hurting the other's feelings. Unfortunately, in the long term it does not resolve the problems of their relationship. If, to put it lightly, smelly feet are the only thing stopping you from having sex, you should persuade your partner to wash his or her feet.

Further problems arise when people experience a genuine headache to avoid sex because they don't want to face up to the issues involved. Men in particular can develop backaches to rationalize subconscious fears of impotence or a belief that they cannot perform well sexually. Rather than be honest with their partners, they suffer real backache. Whether the excuse was originally made consciously or subconsciously is immaterial. After a period of behaving this way, it becomes no longer a white lie but real pain. You may have avoided sex, but you are now also missing work, going out with friends and many other things you want to do.

If you have back pain, for example, it is not an excuse for

avoiding sex. If you say or believe otherwise, you should look beyond this for other reasons. Do you no longer enjoy sex? Do you have marital relationship problems? Do you have fears of no longer performing adequately? If these issues are not addressed, then there is less possibility of overcoming your pain. Many psychologists would say that if these other problems are put right, the pain may no longer have reason for continuing and may perhaps lessen or disappear completely.

It remains a fact that sexual activity can be uncomfortable for chronic-pain sufferers, but most people go on because they consider it important. The discomfort it causes is worth it. Pain isolates people and pulls relationships apart, in some cases destroying them. Sex not only helps to keep a loving relationship intact, but tells your subconscious that you are not giving in to pain's demands.

Most pain problems, whether sexual or concerning day-to-day living, have a solution if you search hard enough. Arnold, an elderly patient, lived to bowl. The worst thing about his pain was that it stopped him from taking part in local matches. When teammates phoned to ask why he had not turned up, he told them that his back made traveling too painful. Staying at home and curtailing his social life upset him, until he thought about it more deeply and realized that he was not being entirely honest. The truth was that he had become forgetful with age and the bus company had changed its routes to the bowling alley. He now had to take two buses instead of one and found it confusing. Often, he arrived late for a match or spent hours getting home again.

Arnold obviously did not want to tell his friends that he felt confused and worried about becoming senile, so he used his back pain as an excuse instead. When he discussed this, someone suggested that he persuade one of his friends to give him a lift. He took up the idea and continued to lead an active life. His back pain was not bad enough to prevent him from bowling – it was the other problems that had prevented him from enjoying himself. The lesson of Arnold's tale, like many others, is that when you use pain as an excuse to avoid social relationships, it always comes back to trap you.

Once this problem is resolved, there are many ways to improve your confidence and self-esteem and move toward normal life again.

Talk Back to Your Subconscious

Your subconscious always plays safe, believing that hurt is harm. At the slightest twinge, it reminds you that you are a pain patient and life is miserable. It constantly nags you not to do too much, warns that it is unwise to go out, exercise or lead a normal life. This does not have to be a one-way conversation. When you are in pain, much of your life is spent tuning in to your subconscious, drifting away into useless thoughts and wishing you were well again. You listen passively, as though taking in a radio play. Things often begin to change, however, when you realize that you can talk back. You can broadcast to your subconscious and have just as much influence over it as it has been exerting over you for all these years.

Because your subconscious sees things only in a very simple way that it believes is in your best interests, repetition may reinforce the message that you are going to live your own life. You are no longer in the passenger seat, but behind the wheel. Changing your lifestyle, as we have seen, is the only effective way to convince your subconscious that you mean business. Repeating positive statements to yourself underlines the message.

One effective way to build your self-esteem is by saying quietly that you are lovable and capable. By doing this on waking, sometime during the day and last thing at night, you are sending a message to your subconscious that you are a nice person and that you can accomplish things.

It is important not simply to say the words, but to think positively about what you mean. As you repeat the phrase, think about someone who loves you, what his or her affection means and how capable you are. There are many things we may do well – driving, cooking, writing – that give a sense of achievement. After about two months, less in many cases, what you are saying submerges itself into your subconscious and becomes part of your life.

The technique is not as unusual as it may appear. We all hold conversations with ourselves every day, but rarely in a positive way. More commonly, we say things like, "I can't be bothered," "I'm sick and tired of this" or "I can't see myself doing that," which are all negative feelings signaling our subconscious that we haven't got the energy or determination to do something.

Visualize Success

You are likely to do things only if you can see yourself doing them. For example, you may long to give up smoking, but if you cannot honestly see yourself in a year's time walking around without cigarettes in your pocket, then there is little chance of succeeding.

When you visualize yourself doing something, it is naturally much easier to accomplish when the time comes. In the U.S., top basketball players are encouraged to visualize the ball dropping into the basket to improve their performance. Research has shown that athletes who play their sports in their minds become better at it more quickly than those who do not.

When you are in pain, negative thoughts are not easy to stop. Instead of tuning in to them and becoming more downcast and anxious, you should cut them off by saying a command to yourself. It may be "Cancel" or "Stop" – anything appropriate will do – and the effect can be surprising.

The problem with negative thoughts is that if you are, say, angry, they can go around and around in your head for hours. It becomes difficult to think about anything apart from how angry you feel or how unfair life has been. You may feel guilty about something you have said and then feel angry for feeling guilty and so on. Unless you firmly stop such thinking, you can spend a whole day like this.

Negative thoughts are a waste of time and energy because they are not actually going anywhere. It is much easier to tell yourself, "Stop. I'll perhaps think about that tomorrow."

Both negative and positive thoughts are very powerful and have great bearing on the way we perceive ourselves. A therapist asked patients to describe themselves in terms of a tree, which allows scope for imagination and can be quite revealing. One man with spine problems described an old oak, hollow and rotten in the middle and barely able to stand. This was the way he felt negatively affected by his pain and, as a result, the way in which he saw himself.

The therapist then asked the patients to visualize an acorn dropping from this tree and the way it would grow. She talked of straight, firm shoots, healthy foliage and branches reaching skyward as the tree became taller and stronger. As she spoke, patients taking part in the exercise visibly straightened and sat more upright as they visualized the tree. The power of positive thought can have a marked effect on both our actions and our feelings.

Turn Down the Volume on Others
People with chronic pain often dwell unnecessarily on remarks other people make. This is partly because pain erodes their

confidence and makes them feel vulnerable. Often the remark is unintentional, but occasionally it can be quite deliberate and very cutting. If you work to rebuild your self-esteem it is important to realize that no matter what anyone says or does to you, you are still a worthwhile person. Once you convince yourself – and your subconscious – that you are lovable and capable, the hurt of chance remarks diminishes. Your own belief in yourself deflects them like a shield.

How to Handle Fear of Failure

When you set yourself targets to change your life, it is natural that you may worry about succeeding. After all, you are attempting things that pain may have prevented you from doing for years. Once this happens there is a tendency for your mind to dredge up all your past failures and parade them one by one until you feel genuinely afraid of going on or pushing yourself further.

One way to overcome this is to turn the emotion to your advantage. As far as your body is concerned, in terms of responses and chemical changes there is very little difference between fear and excitement. It is only a small step from feeling afraid of new challenges to facing them with excitement and anticipation.

Success or failure may depend on exactly what type of thoughts you allow your mind to assemble. Looking back on a Wimbledon defeat, the great tennis player Martina Navratilova reflected that had she remembered all her past successes instead of worrying about failing, she would have won the match.

Past successes are an important part of sports psychology and business management. People display their trophies to remind them how successful they are. If you achieve the target of going out for the day, buy yourself something to keep to remind yourself of what you achieved. Some people open a bottle of wine to celebrate a success and write on the cork what the occasion was. A drawer full of corks or a mantelpiece of mementos can be as much a morale booster as a case crowded with silver trophies.

Of course people fail too. But every failure is an experience that generates success. If you cycle around a corner too slowly, you will probably fall off your bike, but next time you will remember and do it perfectly. People who never take a risk because they are frightened of failing might as well remain in bed.

The more risks you take, the more likelihood there is that your life will change, your pain diminish and your relationships with others be restored to a happier, more fulfilled level.

Healthy relationships help you fight pain

- Keep as interested and involved with people as possible. Try not to let your pain cut you off from others.
- Tell your family and friends what you are trying to accomplish.
- Get them to encourage your healthy behavior.
- Try to keep as independent as you can and not let other people do things for you because of your pain.

EIGHT

Using Your Doctor Wisely

The appointment you have been waiting for finally arrives. The doctor sits behind the desk, pen poised, stethoscope at the ready, eager to help in any way possible. What should fill the next five minutes is a useful two-way conversation in your best interests. But how often does it work that way?

Some chronic-pain sufferers seem to be at war with their doctors as well as at war with their disabilities. Without a positive attitude, five minutes in the doctor's office becomes a combat zone – a situation that is not to anyone's advantage. This sometimes occurs when chronic-pain patients are fed up that their unpleasant symptoms continue unabated without help, or feel frustrated if they think their doctors do not believe them. It is easy to become obsessed with problems of this kind.

On the other side of the desk, from the doctor's point of view, it can be equally frustrating and distressing to have someone describe symptoms that you are unable to help. Sometimes the chronic-pain sufferer seems to make appointments week after week, demanding treatment that is simply not available.

Getting along with doctors and getting the best from them is a two-way process. When you see them they obviously do not have a great deal of time to spend with you. It is best to think out what you are going to say in order to use the time wisely, to your greatest advantage.

Decide on the most important points you wish to get across. Primarily, your doctor needs a brief history of your symptoms and some idea of your main worries. Don't be unfair by bringing up a significant problem right at the end of the appointment, when he or she is running late. If you wrote down some points ahead of time, fine, but remember, he or she is your doctor, not your biographer!

Patients differ enormously. From a doctor's viewpoint, we see some people who offer little information and resent being asked about their problems, while others volunteer so much that no time remains to talk about their problems. The onus is not entirely on you – a good doctor will be able to direct the interview, asking questions that obtain the maximum amount of information from you.

Be prepared for your first visit

To help you get the maximum benefit from your appointment, if you have chronic pain, it is useful to have an idea of what the doctor is likely to need to know from you. Here are some usual questions.

- When did the pain start?
- Why did it start?
- Did it come on gradually, or was it the result of an accident, a burst of unaccustomed activity or some other sudden onset?
- What did you think about it when it first appeared, and what did you do about it?
- Was it bad enough to seek medical advice, or did you wait to see if it got better by itself?

If you have had your condition for some time and are worried about it, you may feel you require a second opinion. Your doctor may already have suggested this anyway, and arranged for a specialist to see you. If not, it is quite reasonable for you to ask for a second opinion if you think it would be relevant.

Doctors have to refer you for a second opinion only if they feel it is medically indicated. They certainly do not have to go on referring you to specialists if none seems able to help. There is a law of diminishing returns, and the more doctors you see, the less likely each one is to be able to do anything for you.

A Typical First Visit

Your physician will want a brief history of the pain, together with the most significant factors that have influenced it. Even though the pain is important to you, it is not necessary to go into great detail. A succinct comment such as "I had some physiotherapy, but it wasn't helpful for more than a few days" is more useful than a blow-by-blow account of everything the physiotherapist did.

No matter how casual the visit may appear, doctors have an agenda they work through to obtain as much information as possible. They will want to know, for example, how the pain has changed, if at all, over the days, months or years it has been present. Has it spread or diminished in the area it affects? Has it changed its nature or its severity?

They will, of course, also want a description of the type of pain it is. Some people find this difficult to put into words. If you have trouble expressing yourself in this way, look at some of the descriptions in the McGill—Melzack Pain Questionnaire in chapter 6 and try to work out from them which are applicable to your type of pain.

When doctors know where the pain is and what type of pain

it is, they will try to discover whether it is constant or variable: does it come in short bursts, and if so, is it caused by specific factors? If it is constant, is it worse at any particular time, such as in the evening, during the night or first thing in the morning? Then they will want to know what things make it worse or better. Again, stick to significant points, not minutiae from several years ago.

If your family physician is hearing about your chronic pain for the first time, he or she will probably already know something about your background. A specialist, however, will probably need to find out a little more about you and your family and the effect the pain has had on your activities and your personality. For example, has it gotten you down or made you frustrated? Has it stopped you from sleeping? What other effects has it had on your life?

Following this, the doctor may do an examination. This is not always helpful in chronic pain; often, the history is the most relevant aspect and will suggest the type of condition that is producing and maintaining the discomfort. However, a brief examination might show if there is any nerve involvement, or how much muscle spasm there is. Depending on the results of the examination, the doctor may decide to refer you for tests.

Treatments Available for Chronic Pain
In medicine, the main aim is to treat the underlying condition. This may be by prescribing antibiotics to kill the bacteria causing a sore throat; or removing the appendix to relieve the pain of appendicitis. For people with chronic pain, the underlying condition is obviously not treatable. However, there are five different types of therapy to reduce discomfort. The most appropriate methods to help the chronic-pain sufferer are selected and then the patient is monitored to see if the treatment is effective.

Because, as we have said, it is unlikely that a cure will result, treatment is aimed at reducing the pain, increasing activity and improving the quality of life. The six types of therapy are:

- medications;
- surgery (which includes permanent nerve blocks);
- temporary nerve blocks;
- stimulation techniques;
- physical treatments;
- psychological techniques.

It is important to look at these in more detail.

Medications

These are so important that a chapter has been devoted to them. Generally, the rule is that nonaddictive drugs can be used, as long as they do not produce side effects. Addictive drugs, such as codeine and oxycodone, should be used only if the sufferer shows signs of increased activity when taking them.

Surgery and Permanent Nerve Blocks

Anesthetists became involved in pain relief through their use

Overuse of drugs

Careful judgment is needed in administering drugs to relieve pain and improve a patient's quality of life. High drug dosages may sedate you, temporarily reduce pain and lessen the likelihood of your complaining, but they do not do you any service.

It is like the story of the camel's hump. A man who thought camels looked uncomfortable with humps bred and crossbred them until the hump had been eliminated. He was pleased with his work, until someone pointed out that he had certainly done an effective job – but they weren't camels anymore. Overuse of drugs may change your personality; you may not complain of pain, but you may no longer be the same person.

of nerve blocks for the relief of postoperative pain. Because nerve blocks gave excellent results for short periods, surgeons and anesthetists thought that more permanent blocks could achieve long-term results with chronic pain.

Severing or surgically damaging a nerve, however, leads to problems. One obvious drawback is that there is a loss of sensation and power and the patient may not be able to feel or move part of his or her body. However, some people would trade this for pain relief.

Unfortunately, damage to the nerve tissue leads to changes in the central nervous system itself, with unpleasant consequences. The remaining fibers of a damaged pain nerve are still able to fire off warning messages to the brain that something is amiss, producing an unpleasant pain in a numb area. This is precisely what happens in conditions such as shingles (postherpetic neuralgia). It can occur either immediately following the block or several months later.

Another problem with chronic pain is that most people experience pain over quite a wide area, supplied by many different nerves. Thus, many different procedures would have to be carried out to reduce the pain in the first place.

However, there are a few conditions for which nerve blocks can be very useful. These include certain types of cancer pain, in specific areas, and trigeminal neuralgia. This is a very painful condition of the face with intermittent, sharp, shooting pain triggered by light touch, a breath of wind or the motion of eating. The trigeminal nerve is susceptible to blocking and a procedure is carried out to burn the nerve. This leaves part of the face numb, but does not produce any disfigurement and completely relieves the pain for long periods. The procedure is appropriate only for trigeminal neuralgia and does not work for other types of facial pain.

Other Surgical Procedures

In the past, many types of surgery have been used on the spinal cord and the brain to try to relieve chronic pain. Unfortunately, the treatment sometimes appears to have been worse than the disease.

The frontal lobes of the brain used to be removed in the 1930s, in what turned out to be a mutilating operation that destroyed the patient's personality. *Lobotomies* are now condemned by most specialists. There are modifications of this type of surgery that cause less damage, but they are very specialized and useful only in one or two rare conditions.

Operations can also be carried out on the spinal cord to relieve pain. One of them, the *anterolateral cordotomy*, interrupts the pain tracts in the spinal cord, but this is generally used only for cancer pain. The pituitary gland used to be surgically damaged for cancer as well, by inserting a needle through the nose into the pituitary and injecting alcohol or other toxic substances. This technique has now been superseded by medication to achieve the same effect with less trauma. In general, surgery on the brain, the spinal cord and nerves to relieve pain is highly specialized and appropriate only in certain limited conditions.

Temporary Nerve Blocks

Treatment may also involve *temporary* nerve blocks being carried out. In many cases, they are diagnostic blocks, with local anesthetic, to try to identify which group of nerves is causing the problem. The sympathetic nerves, for example, can be blocked off for a few hours, and if the pain is relieved, we know that the sympathetic nerves are causing it. Specific spinal nerves can be blocked too, along with the nerves around the facet joints and the intercostal nerves below the ribs.

If you receive temporary nerve blocks you may be given

therapeutic substances, such as steroids or cortisone, combined with local anesthetic. Long-acting steroids can be injected into a joint or into the epidural space, near the spinal cord, to produce an intense local anti-inflammatory effect, reducing the amount of pain and muscle spasm. The importance of this is not that it cures the condition, but that it may break the cycle of spasm and inactivity that keeps the pain going. The pain sufferer will hopefully then be able to become more mobile and relaxed. In a few weeks or months, by the time the effect of the block wears off, the increased strength, mobility and flexibility of muscles will have taken over, affording less discomfort and the freedom to move more easily. Other drugs used in this way include guanethidine to block the sympathetic nerves and hyaluronidase to break down scar tissue.

Stimulation Techniques

Acupuncture

Acupuncture is now such a standard technique for treating pain that it is no longer considered "alternative." A description of acupuncture methods can be found in chapter 9.

Acupuncture stimulation seems to affect the spinal gate, which selects the number of pain messages passing along the spinal cord on their way to the brain. Acupuncture is a high-intensity/low-frequency treatment – high-intensity because you know it is being done and it can even be slightly unpleasant; low-frequency because stimulations are about two per second.

TENS

Another form of electrical stimulation is *transcutaneous electrical nerve stimulation* (known as TENS). This is low-intensity (it doesn't hurt and produces just a tingling sensation) and high-frequency (stimulation is about 100 times per second). When the gate control theory was published by Melzack and Wall in 1965, it was realized that electricity had a part to play in reducing pain. If touch fibers could be stimulated, the resulting messages passing into the spinal cord would "jam" the pain messages. Input of this type actually seemed to close the pain gate.

In electrical nerve stimulation, black carbon electrodes are placed on the skin, usually upstream of the pain. Electrode jelly, or jelly pads, are used to ensure good contact and to avoid burning the skin. A current is then generated from a battery-powered unit. It produces tingling sensations on the skin beneath the pads which sometimes spread between the pads. For the best result, the tingling must mix in with the pain and produce a pleasant substitute for it.

Pain clinics often instruct patients in the use of these machines and may lend them a unit for a time. Because they cost in the region of $140 upward in the U.S., and close to $300 in Canada, and they help only 30 to 40 percent of people who have them, an impulse purchase is not recommended. In any event, the best results come from being taught how to use

Whatever's old...

Like many things in medicine, electrical nerve stimulation is a rediscovery of long-known principles. The ancient Greeks used a similar method with electric eels to relieve the pain of headaches and gout. Documents prepared by the physicians of the period show that significant care was taken to select the appropriate type of fish for the pain.

Hand-generated electricity was used to relieve pain and cure disease in the 19th century. It became so popular that Victorians regarded it as a cure-all, and exaggerated claims were made about its efficacy. They became so bizarre that eventually the use of electricity fell into disrepute. Almost a century later, the gate control theory demonstrated that there was a physiological explanation for the use of electricity, and if applied correctly for the right type of condition, it might be an appropriate and harmless treatment.

the machine properly by someone familiar with them. In general, the more time and effort are spent working with the machine, the more likely it is that good results will ensue.

Different forms of stimulation may be applied with the machine to discover which is most effective. Trial and error reveal the most beneficial position of the pads, and obviously the pain area needs to be fairly localized to give the technique a chance to work. Total body pain is unlikely to be helped by TENS.

If two or three different areas are affected, then units that contain two pairs of leads are used so that different areas can be treated simultaneously. Providing that plenty of jelly is used and the pads are not left on for too long, equipment from reputable companies is quite safe. (Some new electrodes are self-adhesive and require no jelly.) The pads should not be used in the neck region or if you have a pacemaker.

The equipment should also not be used while you drive or operate machinery, at least not until you have had a great deal of experience with TENS. Movement is likely to make the pads shift position, causing a surge of electricity that may produce a sharp sensation, making you jump or lose concentration! However, many patients who are familiar with the system are able to use the machines even while driving.

Electrode Implants

Some patients with TENS machines say that they help up to a point, but feel that they are not powerful enough or do not reach a wide enough area. These people may benefit from an implanted *dorsal column stimulator*. This is an electrode that is implanted surgically in the epidural space, near the spinal cord. A receiver left under the skin picks up signals using a box similar to the TENS machine, and an aerial. This high-tech form of treatment is suitable only for certain types of pain and certain types of people. It needs to be evaluated very carefully before being used.

Electrodes can even be implanted in the brain to stimulate relevant areas, in the hope of reducing pain messages. This technique is clearly even more potentially dangerous than dorsal column stimulation. Although it has proved popular in parts of the U.S., a very thorough assessment of the likelihood of success has to be made before embarking on this expensive and time-consuming method of treatment.

It should be noted that all these stimulation techniques involve cooperation from the patient, and TENS in particular is very much a self-help operation. None of them actually removes the pain altogether, but they do reduce it to more bearable levels. All of them depend on your using this respite to increase activity, with subsequent improvement in your well-being, reduction in muscle spasm and a return to a more normal lifestyle.

Physical Treatments

These include all the physiotherapy treatments many chronic-pain sufferers have had, as well as manipulation, which is dealt with under Chiropractic in the next chapter.

Vibration, local massage and application of heat and cold have all been used to try to reduce chronic pain. Like many treatments, they often have a part to play in cutting down pain, but all depend very much on the patient's personal response. In our experience, none of them works with passive people who are not prepared to do something for themselves. Any that help, however, are worthwhile considering, in conjunction with the self-help techniques outlined in this book.

Psychological Techniques

Hypnosis is now used quite regularly by doctors and can be

useful for chronic pain, though the effect tends to wear off. *Biofeedback* is popular in the U.S. and has been used to treat a wide variety of pain syndromes. The most common technique is to use a device that measures muscle tension, with a dial or indicator that people can watch. They are then encouraged to relax their muscles and observe the results. Usually, more muscle tension is produced on the first attempt and, with practice, better relaxation is achieved. The name comes from the "feedback" of a biological measurement.

Cognitive therapy studies the person's thoughts and feelings about pain and tries to influence them. For example, sufferers are encouraged to think of their pain as a sensation, to realize that it is not harmful or dangerous and to gain a measure of control. Techniques such as these are clearly useful in any form of self-help program.

Behavioral therapy concentrates not on the pain but on what the person does when the pain is felt. The method has been used in the U.S. for 20 years or more and is often a fairly tough program. The therapist draws up a written contract with the patient specifying goals the person wishes to achieve, what he or she will have to do to achieve them and what the staff will do to assist. Steps are taken to withdraw medication, and any exhibitions of pain behavior are ignored. The families are also involved, and are taught to reinforce healthy behavior and to ignore pain behavior. Pure behavioral programs of this kind are now quite rare, although elements of them have become an important part of many treatment regimes and self-help programs.

Be Honest with Your Physician
Many of the treatments described are available only after your family physician refers you for more specialized therapy. Many doctors do not understand the complexities and ramifications

of chronic pain, and feel daunted by the prospect of long-term patients who visit them again and again in the hope of relieving their condition.

It is important to maintain a good relationship with your doctor or specialist to ensure that you get the right treatment for your condition. Chronic-pain patients who devote their lives to searching for a cure waste energy that could be put to more profitable use helping themselves.

If, for example, you continue to visit an orthopedic surgeon following back surgery, and you insist long enough, you are likely to have a second operation. To someone who has a hammer, the saying goes, everything looks like a nail. Despite the fact that there is only a 1 percent chance of further back operations being successful, you may nevertheless force the specialist into operating in the hope of being part of the fortunate 1 percent. If the surgery only makes the problem worse, and you are one of the 99 percent, you will obviously not be very happy. Neither, to an extent, will the surgeon, but at least he or she will have fulfilled his contract and discharged his or her responsibility. The surgeon may have hammered your nail, but it has done no good whatsoever.

The same applies to prescriptions. You know that prolonged use of drugs is not good for you, but when your body demands drugs, you need to obtain them without feeling bad about it. Many chronic-pain patients have a conversation with their physician that goes something like this:

Patient: I don't want to take drugs, but the pain is terrible.

Doctor: I'm sorry, but if that's what you want, there's nothing I can do. You'll have to cope with it.

Patient: I can't possibly cope with it. It's awful.

Doctor: I can give you some pills that might help.

Patient: They were wonderful last time I had them. Thank you.

The doctor writes out the prescription and the patient tells his or her family and friends, "I didn't want to take drugs, but the doctor made me."

If you keep in mind what will genuinely help you to overcome your pain, and phrase your questions intelligently, you will get the best from your doctor. However, if you use your five-minute appointment to complain and pester him or her about your pain, inevitably you will get drugs and advice to rest. This, of course, is the wrong approach to chronic pain, but the fault probably lies more with the way you framed the question than with your doctor.

If you say, "Look, doctor, we both know I'm in pain, but I want to lead a better life. I don't want to take pills and I don't want to give up exercise. Is it safe to carry on?" your physician will be understanding and sympathetic. Ultimately, doctors want to do the best they can for their patients. If you force them to do otherwise, they will capitulate because they have a waiting-room full of other patients who require their attention.

Pressing for what you or your subconscious regards as the easy way out is not necessarily best for you, physically or emotionally. In my own practice, it is not unusual for patients to say to me, "I've been doing my exercises every day, doctor, but that particular one is really too painful. I can't manage it." They phrase it this way hoping to hear me sympathize and advise them to drop the exercise in question. To their great disappointment, I encourage them to carry on and try to break through the emotional barrier, because we both know that for chronic-pain patients hurt does not mean harm.

Using your doctor wisely means being honest, not using him or her for an ulterior motive. Your doctor is on your side, but if the meeting becomes a contest of wills and you pressure him or her into a position that is against your best interests, your relationship will deteriorate. By the time your next appointment comes around, there is every likelihood that your discomfort will have increased and your doctor will get the blame. Dissatisfaction leads to doctor shopping, which, in the long term, will only prolong pain, not reduce it.

NINE

Alternative Medicine

Despite increased amounts spent on conventional health care every year, people are turning to alternative medicine in greater numbers. Doctors themselves have become more aware that certain techniques play a part in helping people with illness. Some therapies, once on the fringe of established medicine, are now so accepted that they can hardly be thought of as "alternative" at all. Relaxation techniques and hypnotherapy are today commonplace in psychiatric units and pain relief centers. Acupuncture is certainly more accepted by the medical establishment than it used to be. Aromatherapy, osteopathy and chiropractic scarcely raise an eyebrow among most physicians, where once they were greeted with skepticism.

So why are more and more people seeking out alternative remedies for their illnesses? On the surface, it might be thought to indicate that modern medicine is not effective, but this is patently not true. Modern drugs and surgery are becoming more reliable, with fewer side effects and higher success rates every year. People do worry about the side effects of medicines and surgery, and the medical profession takes note of their views and tries to improve the quality of life of patients, as well as to reduce their suffering.

Perhaps the answer is that people have a greater expectation of good health. Certainly, increasing numbers expect their physicians to listen to accounts of their symptoms and provide something to relieve the burden of their illnesses. This is understandable in a world where TV advertisements assure us that there is no need to suffer headaches because drug X will magic them away, or drug Y can banish hay fever without ill effects. Advances in medicine tend to be reported sensationally, with little attention to the small print of the research or to any side effects a new treatment might bring. Increased leisure may have given us more time to think about our bodies. But perhaps we worship them too much, without putting in the effort to keep them in good condition.

Tried and True or Hocus-Pocus?

Many folk remedies have been around for thousands of years, and have been used by the general population for centuries, the only change being that they have perhaps become more formalized. Once, people might have consulted their corner druggist or the wise old woman down the street for a non-specific remedy. Now they are more likely to have heard of the fellow across town who practices rolfing, or the woman with a reputation in reflexology.

How effective are alternative remedies, and more important, do they actually work? Obviously, some achieve better results than others, and several different factors have to be considered.

The Placebo Effect

With any form of therapy there is a *placebo effect* (*placebo* is

Latin for "I will please"). From time to time, any normal person may experience the placebo effect, and patients sometimes improve despite a lack of any active treatment. If people recovering from surgery are told they will receive a new drug that gives the finest pain control since morphine, 30 to 40 percent will experience good pain relief after the injection and remain comfortable for some hours. The substance administered could be little more than sterile water!

Obviously, some inert treatments offered to patients will have the effect of making them feel better, even if they contain no active ingredient. It might even be argued that this doesn't matter, provided they have the desired effect.

If someone with severe arthritis visits the doctor wearing a copper bracelet and says that the pain has completely disappeared, the doctor would be foolish to put the patient down. The wisest answer would be "Wonderful – as long as it works for you, keep wearing the bracelet." The doctor is hardly likely to recommend bracelets to other arthritis patients, because some might demand a more scientific approach to their problem.

Of course, the alternative therapy being used may have a genuine effect. Some alternative treatments undoubtedly go beyond the placebo and are being used to try to reduce symptoms with a minimum of side effects. It would take a very hard-nosed scientist indeed to claim that no alternative therapies ever had a therapeutic effect beyond placebos. Most researchers freely admit that there is a lot more to nature than we know at present, and that science has only begun to scrape the surface of the world around us.

Listening Helps

One advantage alternative medicine practitioners have is more time to spend with their patients than the average hard-pressed family physician or specialist. The old saying "Time is a great healer" is particularly appropriate when half the battle is airing your symptoms to someone who listens and cares.

Listening to the patient was one of the attributes of the old-fashioned family doctor, in the days when it was described as "bedside manner." In many instances, this was all the doctor had, since medicines in the last century were generally quite dismal. Some of the therapies available plainly did more harm than good and it is surprising that people survived in spite of them.

Doctors today have a wide variety of treatments at their fingertips, but more patients to attend to and less time to spend with them. In many ways the alternative therapist has taken over the old role of listener and counselor.

Alternative Medicine – Pros and Cons

Alternative medicine has both advantages and disadvantages. On the credit side, it is claimed that it does little harm, and, largely, this is true. It also benefits the patient to have a positive outlook and some optimism about the future. The practitioner spends time with the sufferer, good advice may be given and touch is often used to make the person feel cared for. Above all, of course, there is the potential for genuine action and results.

The downside is that any active treatment carries potential harm. Even an innocent herb such as parsley can cause hemorrhage if the dosage is too high. Acupuncture placed unskillfully around the chest can produce a pneumothorax, or punctured lung. Unsterile needles carry an obvious risk of hepatitis or AIDS. Or someone may abandon conventional therapies because of a total belief in alternative therapy, and the wish to avoid any unpleasant side effects of a medication.

Any initial sense of well-being may unfortunately mask the fact that the condition is worsening, until it is too late.

Commencing any new treatment can produce optimism and positive thoughts about the future, but an awareness that it is not working may lead to deepening depression and feelings of despair, with hope of a cure dashed once more.

The potential cost of long-term, ongoing alternative therapy should also be considered, whether or not it is helping. Multiple treatments may give short-term relief of pain but prove to be the straw that broke the camel's back for chronic invalids without adequate sources of income because of their condition.

The intention here is not to dissuade you from seeking alternative help, but to encourage you to consider its disadvantages and pitfalls. Perhaps the most important negative aspect is that people who pursue alternative treatment in the hope of a cure may be tempted to disregard important self-help techniques that are essential to their improvement.

To help guide you through the maze – and minefield – of alternative medicine, here is a directory of treatments sometimes recommended for use in chronic pain, with comments on their efficacy and drawbacks. Treatments are listed alphabetically.

Acupressure

Acupressure is a mixture of massage and acupuncture. Instead of piercing the skin with needles, practitioners use thumb and fingertip massage to put pressure on acupuncture points. There are different schools of acupressure, including shiatsu (see below).

Local stimulation of pressure points can make some painful conditions worse, due to painful nodules in the muscles. On the whole, acupressure is either harmless or may do quite an amount of good. If three or four treatments fail to help, further therapy is unlikely to be useful. If one treatment makes you worse, then it would be best to abandon it.

One of the great potential benefits of acupressure is that, if it does help, chronic-pain sufferers can stimulate the points themselves, or get a friend or member of the family to help them.

Acupuncture

This Chinese method of treatment has been around for three or four thousand years. The word comes from the Latin *acus*, "a needle," and *punctus*, "a pricking." Acupuncture is thought to have originated when it was noticed that soldiers wounded in battle with arrows and spears appeared to feel less pain than their injuries would suggest. In addition, they sometimes recovered from other ailments.

Treatments were refined over the years by trial and error before acupuncture arrived at its present form. It was introduced to the West by a 17th-century Dutch physician, and in 1823 the British medical journal *The Lancet* reported its successful use in treating rheumatism. Acupuncture's popularity revived in North America and Britain in the early 1970s, when China opened up and many Western physicians observed its use as an anesthetic and pain-relieving agent.

How Does Acupuncture Work?

The Chinese believe that there is a balance in the body between two universal forces or principles known as yin and yang, and that there are 14 meridians extending like trunk roads over the body, each linking acupuncture points.

Acupuncturists follow different schools of diagnosis and treatment but the method is usually the same: a very fine needle is inserted into the relevant points and stimulated, either by twisting with the fingers or by means of a lead clipped to the needle, which is then stimulated by an electro-acupuncture device. (Laser acupuncture has also been used, but its benefits remain uncertain.) There is a slight prick when the needle goes in. Stimulation of the needle produces a heavy numbness, or tingling sensation, which can be quite marked at times.

Modern scientists believe that this stimulation produces activity in rapidly acting pain fibers, resulting in the release of endorphins, the body's natural painkillers. There is also evidence to suggest that acupuncture therapy promotes the release of steroids, which can also have a beneficial effect on many painful conditions.

Acupuncture can certainly have a part to play in the relief of chronic pain. But again, if two or three treatments produce no response, then it is not worth persevering with. A reputable therapist should be found once your family physician has confirmed that there will be no untoward consequences from blocking off any pain.

Aromatherapy

This consists of using highly concentrated and scented plant oils and, like many alternative therapies, has probably existed for thousands of years. The oils are available in many shops.

It is best to get someone else to massage them in, though they can also be inhaled or added to a hot bath. Eucalyptus is said to be good for headaches and muscular pain; juniper for arthritis; marjoram for migraine and cramp; and Roman camomile for headaches. Many oils are also recommended for relaxation.

There is no scientific evidence that any one oil is more effective than another, but most patients find aromatherapy treatment positive and beneficial. It should be stressed, however, that aromatherapy must be part of an active program and not a passive treatment that allows sufferers to lie down and be cured without any effort on their part. As a reward after someone has achieved a target in physical therapy, or to help relaxation in the early stages, it should certainly be of benefit.

Auricular Therapy

This form of acupuncture is practiced by many general acupuncturists. Therapists believe that each part of the body is represented by a point on the ear and various conditions can be improved by stimulating the relevant point with an acupuncture needle, or a small tack or press needle, taped in position in the ear.

There is no evidence that the treatment is any better than acupuncture. A potential advantage is that if a press-stud is used, patients can stimulate the point themselves between visits to the acupuncturist, perhaps intensifying the treatment and reducing cost.

Autogenic Training

This series of six mental exercises is used to relieve stress and help the body to cure itself. In some ways, autogenic training is similar to meditation and yoga. Because relaxation is helpful for chronic pain, it has been used successfully for many people with backache, migraine and irritable bowel syndrome. It is also useful in sympathetic nerve overactivity, and is now so accepted by doctors that it can hardly be called "alternative." However, it should be again stressed that it is unlikely to make everybody with chronic pain completely better, unless used in conjunction with other therapies.

Ayurvedic Medicine

This is the main form of treatment in India, where it is used alongside conventional medical techniques. Its aim is mainly prevention. People keep in touch with a therapist, who monitors their lifestyle and tries to steer them from bad habits that produce illness. When illness does occur, a wide variety of treatments are used, from herbs to mineral supplements to dietary regimes, massage and relaxation. It adds up to a fairly complete way of life that can be difficult for Westerners to adopt if they have been chronically ill for some time. Much of it is common sense, and in keeping with the principles of a pain management program.

Bach Remedies

This form of *homeopathy* (see below) was popularized by an English physician named Dr. Edward Bach. Thirty-eight preparations are made from wildflowers and plants, floated on spring water in sunlight. Chemical analysis of the remedies shows only spring water, with some alcohol. Consequently, most scientists do not accept that there is anything beyond a placebo effect when the remedies produce benefit.

Biofeedback

This technique is now so widely used in North America that it can no longer be regarded as "alternative." Patients are taught to control certain body functions by receiving feedback from a machine that monitors the results of their efforts; the immediate feedback from the machine lets them know when they are succeeding, and when they are not. For example, the machine may monitor their relaxation by measuring skin blood flow in the finger; the blood flow increases as the person becomes more relaxed and blood vessels dilate. Biofeedback can be a very useful way of helping pain.

Chiropractic

A charismatic healer named Daniel Palmer started this form

of treatment in 1895. Scientific trials have shown that manipulation by a qualified practitioner can be very effective for back pain and is worthwhile trying for musculoskeletal pains of any description.

Chiropractors use X-rays to make diagnoses. However, medical practitioners sometimes feel that chiropractors tend to dramatize the underlying problem, saying, for instance, that bones are out of place and need to be manipulated back into position.

Once your physician has ruled out serious, treatable causes for your pain, it is certainly worthwhile visiting a chiropractor, having treatment and repeating it if there is benefit. However, do not attach too much weight to the explanation of the cause of your condition. By all means, carry out the advice to increase your activity, change your lifestyle and relax muscles.

Color Therapy
There is little doubt that color affects mood, but color therapists believe that specific ailments can be cured by adjusting the color input into the body. They may use Kirlian photography (see below) to capture the aura of electromagnetism around the body. Treatment consists of shining colored lights on the patient for about 20 minutes daily.

Color therapy has been used for migraine and various forms of back pain, but it unlikely that it has any inherent value, apart from its effect on mood, relaxation and the placebo response. It is, however, unlikely to be harmful.

Copper Therapy
Wearing a copper bracelet is often cited as a way of reducing arthritic pain. Some studies claim that a remarkable number of pain sufferers are helped in this way, in the belief that traces

of copper from the bracelet penetrate the skin. There is no scientific basis to this contention, but it is certainly a very cheap and harmless method of treatment. Any patient it works for is encouraged to continue its use.

Electrotherapy

The most useful form of this is the transcutaneous electrical nerve stimulator, described in chapter 8. TENS machines are readily available at most pain clinics and should be used in conjunction with medical advice. There is no place for exaggerated claims, and units should not be bought without a reasonable trial period. Consult your doctor or physiotherapist before buying a unit.

Feldenkrais Method

This fairly recent method of self-help was developed by Moshe Feldenkrais, who used the technique to cure his own knee pain and went on to help family and friends. Others have now been taught how to use the method, which helps people to understand how they move and improves their way of moving. Sessions improve posture, reduce pain in muscles and increase the ability to relax. They also increase range of movement and break the spasm–pain cycle. There are obvious parallels with the Alexander Technique and with tai chi. Once again, the idea of gentle exercise, relaxation, improving posture and positive thinking is very similar to a pain management program.

Healing

Sometimes called "spiritual healing," this technique has been used through the ages. A multitude of different techniques are employed and they can often be dramatic. Many healers do not charge a fee but ask for a donation. The medical profession generally takes the view that healers produce a form of placebo response in the patient. Competent healers who produce good results have a great deal of charisma. They are usually very relaxed and encourage positive thinking. As yet, there is no great body of evidence to suggest that healers can provide anyone with more than a "good bedside manner," but studies continue to investigate the phenomenon, with interesting results. In general, healing can be useful for helping chronic pain and producing positive thinking – as long as the person's hopes are not dashed if treatment is unsuccessful, and sessions do not cost too much. Beware of overdramatic or manipulative therapists or groups.

Herbal Medicine

Herbal medicines have been around for thousands of years, and some have been purified and adopted by the medical profession as the cornerstone of treatment for certain conditions. The foxglove plant yields digitalis, which is used for heart failure. From the poppy come morphine and codeine – still the standard painkillers for postoperative pain and pain arising from heart attack and cancer. A form of ASA (aspirin) comes from willow bark.

It has been estimated that 15 percent of medication prescribed by family physicians is plant-based. Throughout the world, herbal medicine is four times as commonly used as conventional medicine. Both in India (Ayurvedic medicine) and in China, herbal medicine is considered orthodox and dispensed in most hospitals.

Herbalists claim that their medication helps many longstanding conditions. Lavender is said to be good for headaches and rheumatism, and mint is also called effective for headaches and stress. In addition, the herbalist may suggest manipulations such as those performed by an osteopath (see below). Medicines, creams or ointments may be prescribed, which are generally naturally grown preparations of whole plants.

This is where herbal therapy diverges from modern medical opinion: in conventional medicine the active ingredient is identified, purified and served up in exact doses; with herbal medicine, you can never be certain of the exact dose, and the plant may contain additional substances that may or may not be useful.

Most commonly available herbal remedies are harmless but, like all drugs, herbs are not completely safe. Research into the properties of exotic compounds now being discovered in the Amazonian jungle may well produce new drugs.

Homeopathy

Homeopathy was developed by a German physician who believed that naturally occurring substances producing symptoms *resembling* those of an ailment would be able to treat the ailment itself if greatly diluted. Plant and mineral substances are most widely used, soaked in alcohol, then diluted to prepare the homeopathic remedy. Arnica and ipecacuanha are used for back pain, and pulsatilla for headache. Poison ivy extract is recommended for arthritis, backache, sciatica and sprains, as well as depression! Treatments can be bought in health food stores, drugstores or homeopathy shops.

Most doctors point out that little scientific research has been done to show that a homeopathic remedy is any better than an inert substance, such as boiled water. It is difficult to believe that preparations so dilute actually contain any active ingredients, but the preparations are also so dilute that they can do no harm. If you decide to try homeopathy, it is advisable to consult a qualified homeopath before undertaking a course of treatment.

Hydrotherapy

Spas are available throughout the world to help people with chronic disease or to relax and reinvigorate a jaded body. A warm bath is universally helpful to many people with chronic pain. Light exercise in water, with the buoyancy it gives the body, is usually well tolerated even by quite infirm people.

Hydrotherapy must be considered as part of a general regime of increasing fitness and producing relaxation. Any hydrotherapist chosen should be carefully screened to ensure that the person is qualified and experienced. Changing from hot to cold baths should be done with care. The general rule is, if you don't like the treatment, don't have it.

Hypnotherapy

Franz Mesmer, an 18th-century Austrian doctor, popularized mesmerism, which developed into hypnotism. Today, there are highly trained therapists who can undoubtedly produce quite dramatic effects in hypnotic subjects. Once the therapist has induced a trancelike state, positive suggestions are given. These are thought to go directly into the subconscious, which has the ability to do a great deal of good to the body if it wishes.

People who are successfully hypnotized can have their pain reduced by a significant degree, although this relief does not always last once the trance is over. For pain, it is better if subjects are taught self-hypnosis so that they can help themselves in the future.

Hypnosis is without doubt a powerful tool. It can be effectively used for chronic pain, but is very time-consuming as a treatment and can be quite expensive. Most doctors share the experience that hypnosis can work at first, but that the effect wears off with time. To maintain it, the subject often needs to continue to work for a considerable period every day, either with the hypnotist, at increasing expense, or with self-hypnosis. On the whole, hypnosis is safe, as long as it's used by a responsible practitioner.

Kirlian Photography

This therapy involves taking photographs of the subject, full-body or specific areas of the body, to reveal an electromagnetic field. The photos are used as a diagnostic tool and a variety of treatments are then instituted in an effort to make the electromagnetic field more "normal." The pictures are certainly dramatic, but they are clearly not a reliable means of diagnosis. Some patients become alarmed at suggestions made by practitioners about the underlying cause of their condition, which sometimes are very inaccurate. For diagnosis, it is better to stick to a qualified doctor.

Massage

Massage has been practiced for more than 5,000 years and takes many different forms that can be helpful in relieving pain and tension. It does not actually cure any condition, but obviously, if it makes you feel better, it is doing some good. A qualified massage therapist should be found, and this may become expensive. It is perfectly reasonable to attend classes given by someone with experience and then give massage to, or receive it from, a partner or close friend. It is important to use massage as part of a rehabilitation regime, rather than passively accepting that massage alone will make you better. If any massage techniques prove to be particularly painful, they should be avoided.

Meditation

Meditation is another ancient form of therapy, and has been used in the East for thousands of years. Yoga (see below) grew from meditation, and over the years various schools of meditation have evolved, some of which often argue about the "right" method. The general aim is to achieve a tranquil state of mind, and some doctors see it as akin to self-hypnosis or deep relaxation. If not too much time or money is devoted to its pursuit, it can become a useful part of coping with pain.

Osteopathy

This therapy was originated by an American doctor in the late 19th century to diagnose and treat mechanical problems such as low back pain. Because such problems are a common cause of chronic pain, osteopathy is worthwhile investigating. There is a register of qualified osteopaths, and practitioners have to take a four-year degree course at an osteopathic college.

Treatment usually involves manipulation of the affected part of the body. Many people benefit from osteopathy, though overzealous manipulation of a painful area can make things temporarily worse. As in all things, choose your osteopath wisely and take stock of how you are progressing after a short course of treatment. If there seems to be improvement, continue.

Osteopathy often appears to be useful for acute conditions, but the problem in chronic pain is that any useful response to treatment is seldom long-lived. Treatment needs to be repeated at regular intervals and the beneficial effect may even fade with time.

Reflexology

Reflexologists use charts of the feet that represent all parts of the body. Massage of the appropriate zone is supposed to clear energy channels, thus allowing the body to heal. Reflexology has been used for many years in conjunction with acupressure, but was popularized by an American surgeon at the turn of the century. Reflexologists undoubtedly have the ability to relax some people, but it is unlikely that the treatment has any inherent effect on pain beyond this. Some practitioners make extravagant and worrying claims that the patient has hitherto undiagnosed illnesses, which can only be improved by a long and expensive course of treatment.

Rolfing

This recently developed therapy involves massage and mild manipulation. Improving posture and reducing muscle spasm are obviously useful.

Shiatsu

A specific form of massage, shiatsu is practiced in Japan. It is similar in some ways to acupressure and, providing a qualified therapist is used, can be of benefit in many painful conditions. It should obviously not be used if it produces a significant increase in pain or if there is no improvement within a few sessions.

Sound Therapy

This may vary from the use of electronic waves directed at the body to chanting and singing. Ultrasound is, of course, a conventional physiotherapy technique, while chanting is part of many meditation techniques. There does not seem to be any inherent effect beyond the use these techniques may already have.

Tai Chi

A form of flowing movements, combined with relaxation and meditation techniques, tai chi was developed in China in the 11th century. Each individual movement is fairly easy, but requires good balance, flexibility and relaxation. The movements are exact and demand a great deal of concentration.

People of any age can try tai chi, although those with chronic pain find the balance and flexibility difficult to begin with. Great benefit can be obtained from gradual progression. It is certainly well worth trying for anyone in chronic pain, even though not everyone will appreciate the philosophy behind it or be able to carry out some of the more difficult movements.

Visualization Therapy

This treatment is based upon the therapist's asking you to imagine a scene in your mind's eye that is related to your problem. If, for example, you have back pain, you might be asked to imagine your spine as a tree, then to describe what the tree looks like. You might see it as withered or lightning-struck. The therapist will encourage you to change it into a sapling that gradually grows straight and strong and in full health.

This technique is used by many alternative therapists, especially those working on relaxation methods. Visualization is a reasonable way of producing relaxation and reinforces positive thinking. If you can't see yourself as healthy, it is difficult to become healthy.

Yoga

Yoga takes many different forms. Hatha yoga, for instance, concentrates on postures, while raja yoga focuses on mental control. In the past 30 years yoga has become extremely popular. Exercise, flexibility and relaxation are what we are trying to develop in chronic-pain sufferers, so as long as the postures are not overdone, yoga can be very useful for people with chronic pain.

There are a great variety of yoga teachers, some perhaps a little too insistent on exercise, but most people can find someone with whom they feel comfortable. Practiced in a group, yoga can be an enjoyable way to improve your health.

These are the most commonly used alternative techniques that have been recommended for chronic pain. Many emphasize self-help through relaxation and exercise. Precise posture is also important, along with positive thinking. Provided that you find a reputable practitioner, that the technique seems to be helping without any side effects and that you realize it is not a cure but a means of reducing your symptoms and increasing activity, then alternative therapy can be of positive benefit.

T E N

Keeping It Going

For all the happiness mankind can gain
Is not in pleasure, but in rest from pain.
— Dryden

We hope you will feel inspired to continue to fight to reduce your pain to an acceptable level after reading this book. Keeping the momentum going on your own is not easy, and self-help groups may provide valuable encouragement and support.

Ten Commandments for Controlling Pain

In addition, there are tried and tested guidelines that can help prevent a slide back into old pain behavior. Adhering to them means increasing your chances of a return to normal life. Some people work hard to follow the rules more diligently than others. No one has ever claimed that overcoming pain is easy, but the more determined you are to break old habits, the less prominently pain will feature in your life.

These "commandments" are important because they can be

your daily mentor for the future. If you forget about them in six months or six years, you will go back to old pain-dominated ways. You may have taken the ideas of pain management on board mentally, but it takes time to undergo a physical conversion.

The situation, though, is not quite as daunting as it first appears, because the more relaxed and physically fit you become, the easier the guidelines are to keep to. There is no doubt, however, that you still have a long road to travel before attaining a level of movement at which you do not have to consciously remember the ideas outlined in this book.

The Ten Commandments have no particular order of importance or priority, but each one must be absorbed as completely as possible into your new routine.

1. Accept That You Have Pain.

Your doctor and family probably accept that you have pain. By now, you know that it is not particularly useful to talk about it, in the sense of informing everyone that you are suffering. It does not help anyone – not your family, your friends, your doctor, your therapist or, most of all, you.

When other people come to accept your pain, it does not mean that they don't believe you are suffering. You either have pain or you don't. Pain is an emotional experience. Just as you experience happiness or depression, pain is real and there is no question of it being imaginary.

Once you and those around you accept that you have pain, it is important not to waste time shopping for a cure. Many people waste their lives going from doctor to doctor, instead of diverting their energy into positive living. We do not live in a perfect world and there is not yet a cure for everything – especially your own particular pain. If there was, then there is every chance you would not be reading this book. Once you begin to search outside yourself for ways of getting better, the possibility of being disappointed increases. Research shows that it is extremely rare for anyone to find a "cure" by visiting doctor after doctor.

Accepting that you have pain means doing something about it by concentrating your efforts within yourself. Learn to ration the valuable energy that pain tries to drain away from you. If your pain should change, then by all means review the situation with your family physician or specialist. Every few years, it is worth having a chat with your doctor to ask if there are new developments that may improve your condition.

There may be a new carbon fiber implant to cure your bad back but, equally, there is the likelihood that no help is available. If there is a possibility of new treatment, always ask what the risks are, but never channel all your energy into clutching at medical straws.

If your specialist says that he or she is still unable to help you, wondering how you can find someone else who can is not a sensible option. Accepting pain means that you are the only person who can do something about it. If you have been shopping from doctor to doctor for years, this may be your final chance.

2. Set Regular Targets and Goals – and Make Sure You Achieve Them.

Setting targets is very important. To make progress, you must set them regularly, rather than rarely. They can be simple goals, and need not even relate directly to your pain – washing your hair, say, or keeping up your exercises, on walking to the post office to mail a letter. Allocate different targets to different days, and include weekly goals, such as visiting a relative, going to church or taking a walk in the park. The secret of setting targets is never to be vague about them. Decide what you are going to achieve each day and when you are going to do it. A week can quickly slide by in dreams and indecision without anything being attained.

It is good to have long-term targets too – you may, for example, plan to return to work within six months or a year – but never leave them vague and open-ended. Break down each long-term goal and think carefully about what, for instance, going back to work may entail: it may require the ability to sit in a chair for four hours, to walk a certain distance, to be able to lift a certain weight. Build toward your big target by achieving individual goals along the way.

It is also important to avoid extremes. If, on one hand, you fail to set targets, you will never make progress at all; if, on the other hand, you set particularly difficult ones, the chances are that you will fail. It is easy to fall into the trap of being too stubborn or too optimistic and setting yourself tasks that prove impossible to achieve. Failure causes fear and depression, which lead back to the familiar, downward spiral of pain.

Set easy, simple targets that you know you can accomplish and do the best you can. List your goals and work methodically through them. If one or two prove hard to achieve, it can be a good indication that you are adopting the right approach. If you consistently achieve 100 percent of all your targets, you are probably pitching them too low.

The key is to create a balance: each day, set yourself regular goals, but spice them with a few that require extra effort to reach. This kind of "friction" in your daily routine stimulates energy and maintains your interest in recovery. Overcoming obstacles increases self-esteem and improves the quality of life. It helps to vary your targets a little, taking care to ensure that as long as you are prepared to contribute time, effort and willingness, you can be fairly sure of attaining them.

If you find you are failing in more than half your objectives, you may be setting your sights too high or going through a bad period. When this occurs, ease back and concentrate on building a firm foundation of achievement to avoid drifting into depression. Everyone in chronic pain should expect bad patches, but if they occur frequently, rethink your routine, because something is probably wrong.

3. Become Physically Fit – Appropriate to Your Age.

If you suffer from chronic pain, you may have difficulty reaching the level of fitness of an average person of your age. One of the reasons for this is that chronic-pain sufferers believe that their pain is a warning not to do too much and they become more unfit than they otherwise might be. Returning to fitness requires a strong belief that the pain you get when you exercise or are active does not indicate damage. Obviously, if you have broken your leg, the pain you feel when you try to exercise is a useful warning that you are harming yourself. This is the nature of pain and the reason your emotional response to it is to reduce activity. When you push through this barrier, your body and your subconscious turn up the pain to prevent you doing more, because they believe that pain is a useful warning sign. In chronic pain, which has no useful purpose, this is not what you need. Becoming physically fit is more vital and important, and you have to ignore the unnecessary warnings in order to work toward it.

Exercise releases endorphins that help you to cope with pain. As a bonus, the body produces endorphins more readily when you are fit than when you are out of condition. The other benefit is strong muscles and ligaments, which not only support any inadequacies in your bony frame but also even support themselves. If you have torn muscles or fibrous nodules in your muscles and ligaments, they tend to settle down as you exercise. When muscles and ligaments are strengthened by exercise, they compensate and take over the actions of weaker ones.

4. *Continue Relaxation on a Daily Basis – Whatever Else Happens.*

Relaxation does not come naturally to most people in pain, which is why it has to be learned. The worse your condition, the more necessary it is to practice relaxation exercises. Unlike riding a bicycle, which can become a habit quite quickly, relaxation often takes a long time to accomplish successfully. The harder you find it to relax, the more effort you need to put in.

Relaxation is an important part of the new lifestyle you will have to adopt to reduce pain, and because of this, time spent on any kind of "body maintenance" is essential. Many of the world's older cultures embody this idea in one form or another. Indians who practice yoga – a combination of light exercise, relaxation and philosophy – are generally healthier than Westerners and suffer fewer disorders induced by stress and muscle spasms.

As you become more proficient at relaxation, you can spend less time at it. Some people learn how to put themselves in a light trance almost immediately. As time goes on, you can acquire the ability to relax in the most difficult of circumstances.

Relaxation is not just for pain, but for every aspect of daily living. Half an hour spent relaxing each day will give a good return: there is evidence to show that people who relax regularly live longer and more healthy lives.

5. *Take Your Analgesics on a Time Basis, Reducing Them Whenever Possible.*

Simple painkillers are fine as long as you do not suffer side effects. ASA, acetaminophen and anything that can be bought off the shelf (such as ibuprofen, etc.) is quite acceptable – as long as it does not make you suffer in other ways.

When you move up on the analgesic ladder to codeine-based compounds, you should seek advice from your doctor.

It may be better to take such pills according to the clock, not according to the pain. The more often you take them when the pain dictates, the more your brain will believe you need pills when the pain is bad and turn up the pain volume to demand more. Try to dissociate the taking of drugs from the intensity of the pain. If your pain becomes worse, try not to take more pills than you had already planned; otherwise it can be increasingly difficult to break the cycle.

6. Remember and Understand the Psychological Factors Maintaining Your Pain, and What You Can Do to Prevent Them from Making Your Pain Worse.

Because pain is a psychological experience, psychological

The Ten Commandments of pain management

1. Accept that you have pain.
2. Set regular targets and goals – and make sure you achieve them.
3. Become physically fit – appropriate to your age.
4. Continue relaxation on a daily basis – whatever else happens.
5. Take your analgesics on a time basis, reducing them whenever possible.
6. Remember and understand the psychological factors maintaining your pain, and what you can do to prevent them from making your pain worse.
7. Get angry with your pain if it seems to be getting the upper hand.
8. Get your family and friends to reinforce your positive action – not your pain and disability.
9. Remember that working in a group is more fun and more effective.
10. Think positive.

factors will make it worse, keep it going or influence it in some way. The factors differ and vary from person to person.

It may be that the subconscious is maintaining pain for reasons buried in the distant past. Another psychological factor is using pain as an excuse to get out of doing something you do not enjoy. Once you do this, the situation always rebounds on you. People then complain that pain stops them from doing things they enjoy, as well as the things they dislike.

It is important to study yourself and discover exactly what makes the pain worse. Understanding the psychological aspects of your problem can modify your life and help you to accomplish more.

7. Get Angry with Your Pain If It Seems to Be Getting the Upper Hand.

Anger is a negative emotion and has to be handled carefully, but only because we generally use it in the wrong way. It is easy for people to feel angry with doctors, because they have been sold the idea that medicine can make everyone better. They are angry because no one can help them. But there is little point in this. Doctors have not failed because they don't want to help.

Similarly, some people get angry with doctors who have caused them pain. This is understandable, but it too is not useful. Becoming angry, frustrated and tense only makes the pain worse.

People get angry with their families for not understanding enough about them or failing to cope with them. Indeed, one of the worst things about chronic pain is that it makes people irritable. But it is no use getting angry with someone else. You have to train yourself to be more controlled. Rehearse in your mind what makes you snap when your family says something. After all, it is not they who caused your pain.

Most important, never be angry with yourself. When you see other people coping well with their pain and making progress, you should not feel angry about how difficult you find things. We all move at our own pace. The answer is not to feel angry about your lack of progress, but to keep going.

Try getting angry with your pain instead. Focus all your energy on the pain, on the sole thing that everyone dislikes. When you feel your emotions rise, tunnel them into your pain and make your anger shrink it. This can actually be done and is a useful way to channel negative emotions so that they do not rebound off those around you.

8. Get Your Family and Friends to Reinforce Your Positive Action – Not Your Pain and Disability.

Here, we are back to Pavlov's dogs again. Whenever Pavlov gave his dogs a meal, he rang a bell. After a few days the dogs associated the bell with being fed. When the bell rang, they salivated on cue. Once this kind of conditioning behavior is established, you no longer have to reinforce the sound of the bell with food to make the dogs drool. Like many things in life, such as speaking with an accent, it becomes a conditioned response.

When people reinforce your illness, they condition you to being ill. Every time you do something and they step in to help because they think what you are doing will make you ill, they condition you to become an invalid. Continue this for long enough and you will remain an invalid, long after the original problem has gone away.

Your family have to learn to ignore you more kindly, or to help in a positive way by creating time and space for exercise and relaxation. Family and friends should encourage you to be well. If you have been complaining about pain for 20 years and suddenly do something positive, that is the time you should be paid the most attention.

Instead of rejecting your family's offers of help, explain to them that it has to be constructive for you to improve mentally and physically. We all need the support of people around us, but only in the right way.

9. Remember That Working in a Group Is More Fun and More Effective.

It is important to connect with others for exercise and relaxation, as well as for social events. Being alone and in pain isn't much fun. When you have read this book, you may feel that you do not want to associate with others who have chronic pain. Even those who return to work still need a group of some kind to communicate with. It is extremely difficult to sort out some problems by yourself.

The group you join does not have to be a pain group. You can join local classes for exercise or yoga. The important thing is that if you do not turn up for two weeks, someone will probably phone and ask if you are all right or encourage you to return.

Social contact is one of the cornerstones of civilization. Isolating yourself is the worse thing you can do. As the song tells us, people need people, for help, advice and encouragement. Whatever exercise or relaxation you plan, always join a group of some kind to keep you going.

10. Think Positive.

This is not easy when the road to recovery often appears to be three steps forward and four steps back. You must be prepared for times when you seem to be making little progress. Avoid sitting around feeling depressed and wondering what went wrong by planning for such occasions. Revise your targets to prepare for the possibility that you may have to rest for a few days.

Giving up and throwing away all the work you have put in, and the progress you have made, is the easy option. No one ever said that achieving a normal life again would be trouble-free. When times are bad, you have to be positive and take pride in all your achievements.

If you work on each of the Ten Commandments you may receive benefit for a short period or a tremendous improvement that remains with you for the rest of your life. Some chronic-pain patients have rebuilt their lives and become more physically active than ever before.

Not everyone can do as well as Mike Spring, who overcame painful paralysis to build his own boat and sail single-handed to the Azores. But there are many unsung pain heroes who quietly rebuild their lives. It is appropriate to conclude with the story of one of them – a 59-year-old man named Arthur, who suffered severe pain below an operation scar for six years. Any walking caused muscle spasm and made Arthur's pain worse. He was unable to play golf or to follow his hobby of gardening because he could not dig. Intensive treatment had failed to reduce his discomfort and allow him to return to work.

Arthur started on our pain management program in May 1992. He was taking 20 pills of various kinds each day. As well as having difficulty in walking, he could not climb stairs, was unable to sit for more than a few minutes and found concentration almost impossible.

At the start of the program Arthur realized that the object was not to get rid of his pain, but to learn how to live with it. He took the idea on board and pressed himself into forming a firm opinion that *"this will work."*

He stopped taking his pills and soon felt considerably better. After just one week his quality of life had improved enormously. His thinking became positive, and within a short time he felt that he had his life under control again. The pain was no longer getting the better of him – he felt that he was finally in charge of the way it affected his life.

After the program, he did not feel a need for drugs, and his thinking was much clearer. He felt far less moody, could move around better and actively enjoyed his new lifestyle.

Arthur still does exercises every day and puts aside a period for relaxation, which he now finds easy to do. His pain has certainly not gone away, but he is confident of having more control of its effect on him. Arthur also discovered that, as you become older, your body changes and it is not unusual to have aches and pains. He feels it is important not to confuse the two and to blame all your shortcomings on chronic pain.

He has since returned to work, climbs stairs and plays golf regularly. The pain is still there, but he now has a quality of life that was not present before.

Arthur's success story is the kind we expect of people who follow the advice outlined in this book. With the right attitude, the future is not bleak. The opportunities are there and the possibilities enormous – provided you have the hope and the will to keep going.

Best wishes for success.

Table of Drug Names

Generic name	Some common brand names
Painkillers	
Acetaminophen	Atasol, Tempra†, Tylenol
ASA (aspirin)	Bayer, Bufferin, Entrophen†
Anti-inflammatories	
Diclofenac	Voltaren
Diflunisal	Dolobid
Etodolac	Lodine*, Ultradol†
Flurbiprofen	Ansaid, Froben†
Ibuprofen	Advil, Motrin†, Nuprin*
Indomethacin	Indocid†, Indocin*
Ketoprofen	Orafen†, Orudis
Mefenamic acid	Ponstan†, Ponstel*
Naproxen	Anaprox, Naprosyn, Naxen†
Piroxicam	Feldene
Propoxyphene	Darvon*
Sulindac	Clinoril
Tenoxicam	Mobiflex†
Tiaprofenic acid	Surgam†
Tolmetin	Tolectin
Narcotics	
Acetaminophen + codeine	Empracet†, Emtec†, Phenaphen, Tylenol with Codeine
Acetaminophen + oxycodone	Oxycocet†, Percocet, Roxicet, Tylox*
Anileridine	Leritine†
ASA (aspirin) + codeine	222†, Emcodeine*
ASA (aspirin) + oxycodone	Percodan
Hydromorphone	Dilaudid, Hydromorph Contin†
Morphine	M-Eslon†, MS Contin, MSIR, Oramorph, Statex†
Pentazocine	Talwin
Tranquilizers	
Chlordiazepoxide	Librax†, Librium*
Diazepam	Valium
Lorazepam	Ativan
Antidepressants	
Amitriptyline	Elavil†, Etrafon
Desipramine	Norpramin
Nortriptyline	Aventyl, Pamelor*
Trazodone	Desyrel
Venlafaxine	Effexor
Miscellaneous	
Carbamazepine	Tegretol
Gabapentin	Neurontin
Guanethidine	Ismelin
Mexiletine	Mexitil

* Available in U.S. only

† Available in Canada only

Glossary

Acupressure: a technique to relieve pain, consisting of massage and acupuncture.

Acupuncture: an ancient Chinese method of pain relief in which needles are inserted at specific points called "meridians" in the body.

Acute pain: pain that develops rapidly but does not last long. (*See also* **Chronic pain.**)

Analgesic ladder: drug treatment for pain, from simple ASA to codeine and morphine, that increases in strength as you go up the ladder.

Anterolateral cordotomy: a pain-relief procedure that interrupts pain in pain tracts in the spinal cord.

Anticonvulsants: drugs that inhibit or control convulsions or seizures.

Biofeedback: a technique in which patients are taught to control certain body functions by receiving feedback from a machine.

Body language: visual signals your body sends out (gestures, posture, etc.)

Catastrophizing: making problems worse by exaggerating anxieties and fears.

Chiropractic: treatment of pain and disorders through physical manipulation.

Chronic pain: pain that lasts for a long time, or recurs frequently. (*See also* **Acute pain.**)

Cognitive distortions: negative internal conversations.

Dorsal column stimulator: an electrode implanted surgically in the epidural space to control pain.

Electrotherapy: *See* **TENS.**

Endorphins: pain-blocking chemicals produced by the body.

Fast pain: sharp or sudden pain such as that indicating ongoing injury, usually resulting in a reflex action to escape the cause of pain. (*See also* **Slow pain.**)

McGill–Melzack Pain Questionnaire: a test to measure how well someone is coping with pain.

Myofascial pain: a painful muscle condition in which muscles develop tender fibrous nodules.

Nerve blocks: severance or surgical damaging of a nerve to relieve pain.

Neurotransmitter: a biochemical substance that transmits or inhibits nerve pulses.

Nociceptors: nerve cells that transmit unpleasant messages to the brain.

NSAIDs: nonsteroidal anti-inflammatory drugs, including ASA and ibuprofen; situated on the first rung of the analgesic ladder.

Osteopathy: treatment of the body's mechanical problems through physical manipulation.

Pain threshold: the level at which a sensation becomes painful. Pain thresholds are fairly consistent from person to person.

Pain tolerance: the ability of a particular individual to ignore or cope with pain. Pain tolerance varies widely from person to person.

Phantom-limb pain: pain that feels as though it arises in an amputated limb.

Placebo effect: an apparent result (such as pain relief) from an inactive substance, for psychological reasons; people who expect to feel better often do, at least temporarily.

Postherpetic neuralgia: a painful lingering condition following nerve damage from shingles.

Prostaglandins: hormones that irritate nerve endings and help nerve fibers carry pain messages to the brain.

Referred pain: pain felt in some part of the body other than where the cause is actually located.

Secondary analgesics: medications that reduce pain as a side effect, but are used primarily for other purposes.

Slow pain: deep, long-lasting pain, such as that resulting from an earlier injury, often resulting in contraction and rigidity of muscles. (*See also* **Fast pain.**)

Targeting: setting small, achievable objectives to unlearn bad pain behavior and promote positive activity.

TENS: transcutaneous electrical nerve stimulation; electrical stimulation used to relieve pain.

Tranquilizers: drugs used as calming agents to relieve and control certain emotional disturbances, neuroses, psychoses, etc.

Trigeminal neuralgia: a disorder creating severely painful spasms in nerves of the head and face; the cause is unknown.

Visualization: relaxation therapy using the person's own imagination to create positive images.

Further Resources

Organizations

Canada

Acupuncture Foundation of
Canada Institute
2131 Lawrence Ave. E.,
Suite 204
Toronto, ON M1R 5G4
(416) 752-3988

Arthritis Society
393 University Ave.,
Suite 1700
Toronto, ON M5G 1E6
(416) 979-7228
Fax: (416) 979-8366
www.arthritis.ca

Back Association of Canada
83 Cottingham St.
Toronto, ON M4V 1B9
(Please write for info
package.)

Canadian Chiropractic
Association
1396 Eglinton Ave. W.
Toronto, ON M6C 2E4
Toll-free: 1-800-668-2076
Fax: (416) 781-7344
www.inforamp.net/~ccachiro

Canadian College of
Osteopathy
39 Alvin Ave.
Toronto, ON M4T 2A7
(416) 323-1465
Toll-free: 1-800-263-2816
(recorded info)

Canadian Pain Society
1278 Tower Rd.
Halifax, NS B3H 2Y9
www.medicinc.daloca/gorgs
/cps

Heart and Stroke
Foundation of Canada
160 George St., Suite 200
Ottawa, ON K1N 9M2
(613) 241-4361
Toll-free: 1-888-473-4636

Migraine Foundation
365 Bloor St. E., Suite 1912
Toronto, ON M4W 3L4
(416) 920-4916
Toll-free re membership:
1-800-663-3557
24-hour info line:
(416) 920-4917
Fax: (416) 920-3677
www.migraine.ca

North American Chronic
Pain Association of Canada
150 Central Park Drive,
Unit 105
Brampton, ON L6T 2T9
(905) 793-5230
Fax: (905) 793-8781
Toll-free: 1-800-616-7246

U.S.

American Academy of
Medical Acupuncture
5820 Wilshire Blvd., Ste. 500
Los Angeles, CA 90036
(213) 937-5514
Toll-free: 1-800-521-2262
www.medicalacupuncture.org

American Chiropractic
Association
1701 Clarendon Blvd.
Arlington, VA 22209
(703) 276-8800
Toll-free: 1-800-986-INFO
http://www.amerchiro.org/ara

American Chronic Pain
Association
P.O. Box 850
Rocklin, CA 95677
(916) 632-0922
Fax: (916) 632-3208
acpa@pacbell.net

American Council for
Headache Education (ACHE)
875 Kings Highway,
Suite 200
Woodbury, NJ 08096-3172
Toll-free: 1-800-255-ACHE
http://www.achenet.org

American Heart Association
7272 Greenville Ave.
Dallas, TX 75231-4596
(214) 373-6300
http://www.amhrt.org

American Osteopathic
Association
142 E. Ontario St.
Chicago, IL 60611
(312) 280-5800
Toll-free: 1-800-621-1773
http://www.am-osteo-assn.org

American Pain Society
4700 West Lake Ave.
Glenview, IL 60025
(847) 375-4715
Fax: (847) 375-4777
http://www.ampainsoc.org

Arthritis Foundation
1330 W. Peachtree
Atlanta, GA 30309
(404) 872-7100
Toll-free: 1-800-283-7800
(recorded info)
www.arthritis.org

Association for Applied
Psychophysiology and
Biofeedback
10200 W. 44th Ave.,
Suite 304
Wheat Ridge,
CO 80033-2840
Toll-free: 1-800-477-8892
http://www.aapb.org

National Headache
Foundation
428 West St. James Place,
2nd floor
Chicago, IL 60614-2750
Toll-free: 1-800-843-2256
http://www.headaches.org

Books

Alberti, Robert E., and Michael L. Emmons. *Your Perfect Right: A Guide to Assertive Living*. San Luis Obispo, CA: Impact, 1990.

Benson, Herbert, M.D. *Beyond the Relaxation Response*. New York: Times, 1984.

Burns, David D., M.D. *Feeling Good: The New Mood Therapy*. New York: Morrow, 1980.

Caudill, Margaret, M.D. *Managing Pain Before It Manages You*. New York: Guilford, 1995.

Corey, David, M.D., with Stan Solomon. *Pain: Learning to Live Without It*. Toronto: Macmillan, 1988.

Hanson, R.W., and Kenneth E. Gerber. *Coping with Chronic Pain*. New York: Guilford, 1990.

Melzack, Ronald, M.D., and Patrick Wall. *The Challenge of Pain*. New York: Basic, 1983.

Shone, Neville. *Coping Successfully with Pain*. Boston: G.K. Hall, 1993.

Starlanyl, Devin, M.D., and Mary Ellen Copeland. *Fibromyalgia and Chronic Myofascial Pain Syndrome*. Oakland, CA: New Harbinger, 1996.

Index

To the Reader

Your Personal Health Series is developed with the Canadian Medical Association and will encompass more than 20 subjects. The first six publications are *Migraine, Eyes, Arthritis, Sleep, Crohn's Disease & Ulcerative Colitis* and *The Complete Breast Book*. We expect to publish at least three new titles each year.

If you wish to be kept informed about the series, please complete and send us this page (or a photocopy). We will be pleased to send you periodic publication notices on new and forthcoming titles.

Key Porter Books Limited
70 The Esplanade
Toronto, Ontario M5E 1R2 Canada
Telephone (416) 862-777 • Fax (416) 862-2304

☐ Please keep me informed about *Your Personal Health Series*

☐ Please ship and bill ____ copy/ies of each new book upon publication.

_____
NAME

_____
AFFILIATION (COMPANY/ASSOCIATION/INSTITUTION/MEDICAL AFFILIATION)

_____
ADDRESS

_____
CITY/TOWN   PROVINCE   POSTAL CODE

PAYMENT BY: ☐ VISA   ☐ MASTERCARD

_____
CREDIT CARD NO.

_____
EXPIRY DATE

_____
SIGNATURE

☐ Please invoice to above

Publication prices will vary and are subject to change without notice. GST and Shipping & Handling Charges will be added to the invoice.